TWICE AS HARD

TWICE AS HARD

THE
STORIES OF
BLACK
WOMEN
WHO FOUGHT TO BECOME
PHYSICIANS,
FROM THE CIVIL WAR
TO THE 21ST CENTURY

• • •

JASMINE BROWN

BEACON PRESS · BOSTON

BEACON PRESS
Boston, Massachusetts
www.beacon.org

Beacon Press books
are published under the auspices of
the Unitarian Universalist Association of Congregations.

26 25 24 23   8 7 6 5 4 3 2 1

This book is printed on acid-free paper that meets the uncoated paper
ANSI/NISO specifications for permanence as revised in 1992.

Text design and composition by Kim Arney

Library of Congress Cataloguing in Publication Data is available for this title.

Names: Brown, Jasmine, author.
Title: Twice as hard : the stories of Black women who fought to become
physicians, from the Civil War to the 21st century / Jasmine Brown.
Description: Boston : Beacon Press, [2022] | Includes bibliographical references and
index. | Summary: " Black women physicians' stories have gone untold
for far too long, leaving gaping holes in American medical
history, in women's history, and in black history. It's time
to set the record straight."—Provided by publisher.
Identifiers: LCCN 2022043511 (print) | LCCN 2022043512 (ebook) |
ISBN 9780807013373 (paperback) | ISBN 9780807025093 (ebook) |
Subjects: LCSH: African American women physicians—United States—Biography. |
African American physicians—United States—Biography. |
Women physicians—United States—Biography. |
African American physicians—United States—History—19th century. |
African American physicians—United States—History—20th century.
Classification: LCC R153 .B76 2022 (print) | LCC R153 (ebook) |
DDC 610.922—dc23/eng/20220930
LC record available at https://lccn.loc.gov/2022043511
LC ebook record available at https://lccn.loc.gov/2022043512

CONTENTS

SET THE RECORD STRAIGHT

As I sat in my cramped dorm room in Oxford, England, I listened to a voice resonating through my laptop. It transported me to the other side of the world. Back home.

"After I got a taste of this thing of college, then I had to have more of the same . . . I loved it . . . I mean, my getting back to college, I was delighted. Now my only fear there was that I could not possibly make enough money with my mother to go into the next year. So, I decided to make as much of that year as I could, you see. And so that I could at least say that I had two years of college, or three years of college, you see."[1]

The sound of Dr. May Chinn's voice seemed so familiar. It felt as though she was one of my great-grandmothers. Dr. Chinn and I were born a hundred years apart, and she passed away forty years ago. Still, her voice bent through time and touched my soul. I could imagine us sitting on a pillowy couch in a cozy living room, both sipping a hot cup of English Breakfast tea as she told me her life story. She bravely hurdled the challenges of being a black woman entering the unwelcoming field of medicine in the early twentieth century. And she came out on the other side in triumph as a skilled physician who made a huge impact in her patients' lives.

Her story resonated with me. As a black woman medical student who will be the first in my family to become a physician, I've faced my own set of trials. When Dr. Chinn recounted her experience with medical colleagues who disregarded and ostracized her, I felt the burn of salt being rubbed into wounds that have not had the opportunity to heal.

I t was the beginning of my junior year in college at Washington University in St. Louis, and my first day back in my neuroimmunology lab after a few weeks of vacation. I approached the lab's entry door with my ID in hand. An older white man whom I didn't recognize trailed behind me. He didn't provide any explanation about his connection to the lab. I didn't request one. While the lab is large and composed of multiple smaller labs within one space, we have a culture of opening the door for one another. We assume good intent. This is the mindset I adopted as I prepared to give this unidentified man access to my lab.

Swipe. I placed my ID through the card reader, but a red light flashed in response. I reminded myself that this card reader was finicky. So I tried again.

Swipe, swipe. More red light. This time my cheeks flushed to match the color of the reader. It didn't make sense. My card was supposed to work. It had worked all summer. I had even spoken with technology services before my vacation to ensure that my card would still work when I returned for the school year. I was confident that the problem was with the card reader, not my card. So I tried again.

Swipe. Red light blinked back at me in innocence. I relented. Steeped in embarrassment, I asked the mystery man if he would open the door for us.

With raised suspicion, he countered, "Are you supposed to be in this lab?"

Immediately, my body froze. While his question may have seemed innocent, the doubt laced into his words brought me back to my childhood. Since elementary school, other kids have told me that I am stupid and will never belong in the highly praised realms of science and medicine. "You're black. Black people aren't smart."

When my AP calculus teacher announced that I had scored at the top of my class on the midterm exam, my classmates looked at me with shock. I was the only black person in the room. They didn't understand how I could've outperformed them on a test, let alone a math test. Then, as I neared the end of my high school career, people who claimed to be my friends suddenly turned on me. They confidently explained that I would get accepted into college because I was black. Not because I had a near perfect GPA with countless AP classes on my transcript, coupled with the fact that I was president of multiple organizations and a varsity athlete. My academic achievements were worthless in their eyes. The only purpose I served was filling a quota. To make matters worse, numerous classmates told me that I would never succeed in higher education or in a STEM career. I was a black woman, twice disadvantaged. Success was incompatible with my identity.

The mystery man's supposedly harmless question excavated immense pain that I had fought so hard to keep buried. Feeling like a deer in headlights, I answered his question without being able to vocalize the emotions that suddenly rushed over me. "Yes. I'm a student at Washington University, and I work here."

He was not convinced by my explanation. "Can I see your ID?"

I readily handed it over.

"Why doesn't it look like my faculty ID?"

"Because I'm a student. I'm a student at the university."

My ID read "Washington University in St. Louis" at the top and had a recent photo of me in color, with the word "Student" below. After examining my identification, he remained skeptical. The air between us was tense. It was like I was a thief preparing to break into a lab to steal some chemicals. While I wasn't the most strategic—choosing to "break in" during work hours when the lab was filled with other people—I was still a threat. And he was the (still-unidentified) cop ready to right my wrongs. But none of this was true. I was just a college student whose excitement to reenter this beloved space had suddenly transformed into sorrow. He continued his line of questioning, and I continued to answer helplessly. Eventually, he gave up his defense of the lab and opened the door. I followed him in and quickly went to my lab bench.

Soon, I realized that this man worked right next to my lab. His office adjoined the room where I prepared countless specimen trays for qPCR experiments. With my white coat on and my lab notebook in hand, I tried to walk confidently whenever we crossed paths. I wanted to prove to him that I was truly a scientist in this lab, not a thief, while ignoring the queasiness that arose whenever I saw him. After that incident, he never said anything to me again. Never looked me in the eye. Never acknowledged my presence or the pain that he had caused me.

Why did he treat me like that? Why didn't he believe me when I told him that I was a college student working in the lab? The day with the faulty card was the day that I realized I was the only black person in my lab. When I attended research talks in the building, I was always the only black person in the room. It seemed like I was the only black scientist in the entire seven-floor building. And I was only a student! The only other black people I saw working in the building were members of the janitorial or kitchen staff. I guess based on this data sample, it was reasonable for this man to assume that I wasn't a scientist in the lab—even though my photo ID should've been enough proof that I truly was affiliated with the university.

Following the encounter with that man, I no longer felt excited to go to the lab each day. I felt anxious. My fast-beating heart tried to keep my feet from walking to the train station. The smell of urine in the underground station became more repugnant, threatening to induce nausea. The stares I received from people as I shuffled off the train and onto the medical campus seemed more aggressive, echoing the message from the man in my lab: You don't belong here. I felt like I was walking on eggshells. Something was bound to crack.

Then, one day, I was invited to attend a small group session with a visiting Harvard professor, through the John B. Ervin Scholars Program, an organization at WashU that supports students who exhibit leadership potential and a commitment to serving their communities. As a part of our introductions, we were tasked to answer: "What makes you anxious?" Although I typically try not to be vulnerable in large groups, I decided to open up since I knew many of the people in the room. As I retold my experience in the lab, tears rushed down my face. I hadn't realized how much this encounter had affected me. After the meeting, I spoke more about this issue with the dean of the Ervin Scholars Program. As I laid my wounds bare, a weight lifted off my shoulders. I was not in the wrong. And it was okay for me to feel the pain that I felt. My emotions were valid. Suddenly, I felt more comfortable speaking about the incident.

A few weeks later, I presented my research at WashU's Fall Undergraduate Research Symposium. As I stood crowded around a poster with two other black research students, my mind wandered. Sharing this biomedical space with them reminded me that, while I was the only black scientist in my lab, I was not the only black scientist at my university. That realization was followed by another. I was not the only black researcher who experienced microaggressions. Once I was able to look past my individual experience, memories of others' experiences rushed back to me. I had numerous black friends from various academic institutions who had reached out to me for solace after facing their own personal traumas in research environments. I wasn't alone. We weren't alone. So why had these experiences made each of us feel so lonely? These incidents had seemed like isolated events. We were usually the only black scientist in our respective research spaces, so we oftentimes lacked support during these difficult encounters. Each of us wondered if we had done something that warranted the treatment we received. And it was difficult not to defer to the perspective of the person doing the microaggression, since frequently that person held a superior position in the lab. But these were not isolated events. They were recurring problems that signaled much deeper issues within the research community. Because we were typically siloed in different corners of a research institution, it was hard to see this pattern. But now that we were together at this symposium, the problem became vividly clear to me.

This epiphany moved me to act. First, I founded the Minority Association of Rising Scientists (MARS). This organization aims to counteract the detrimental effects of implicit bias and imposter syndrome through programming that promotes community among students of color pursuing research careers. It also brings awareness to the prevalence of imposter syndrome and introduces ways to combat it. Among its events, MARS offered a popular series of meetings where black graduate students spoke about their experiences in science and gave advice on how we undergraduates could be successful in the field. Whenever we had these mentoring sessions, at least one MARS member would tell me how the session helped them with something they were struggling with, either in their current lab or in their pursuit of a research career.

The morning after one of these sessions, I walked over the bridge connecting my apartment to my college campus. I was on my way to an organic chemistry class. While a cold wind brushed against my skin, I was warmed by an energy reverberating from deep inside me. A sensation stronger than butterflies kindled in my stomach. I felt like I was walking toward my purpose. And while working to help others, I was tending to my wounds from the day with the faulty ID card, as well as many other related traumas.

A year later, I received the incredible news that I was selected as a Rhodes scholar. This provided me with a platform to have an even broader impact within the advocacy space. As my professional interests shifted toward medicine, I decided to apply my experience with MARS to tackle a similar issue within medicine. I pursued a master of philosophy in the history of science, medicine, and technology at the University of Oxford. My dissertation focused on the social and structural barriers put in place to prevent black women from entering medicine in the US. I figured that if I could determine the historical underpinnings of the underrepresentation of black women in medicine, I would be better equipped to help increase the number of black women, and other underrepresented minorities, within the field.

Initially, the research and master's classes were extremely draining. I learned how deeply race- and sex-based prejudice ran. For centuries throughout the world, Europeans and white Americans employed tactics to deprive black people of opportunities and deplete their quality of life. When I studied racial dynamics within medicine, I found countless social and structural obstacles meant to keep white men as the dominant group within medicine. It felt like so much was stacked against me as a black woman interested in medicine. At the same time, I struggled to find information on notable black women physicians. Up to that point, I had never met a black woman physician, and I hadn't been taught about any in school. I knew they must exist, but their histories were buried or never properly documented to begin with. I became desperate to find them, to get to know their stories, and to understand what inspired them to become physicians. I needed to know how they survived and pushed forward in the face of so many racist and sexist obstacles.

After more than six months of mining the internet and archives for these women, I finally struck gold. I found an archive at Harvard Radcliffe Institute's Schlesinger Library that included interviews from 1976 to 1981 with notable black women who were in their seventies, eighties, and nineties. There were interviews with a handful of black women physicians in the collection. This is how I discovered Dr. May Chinn. Once I found substantive information about one African American woman physician, she led me to the next, and the next. When I felt my knees begin to buckle under the weight of the knowledge that, for well over a century, people like me had been rejected from medical schools and then residency programs solely because of their identities, these black women's stories were my antidote. They gave me the strength to keep running in my own race toward a career in medicine.

So when I earned my master's degree from the University of Oxford and then began medical school at the Perelman School of Medicine at the University of Pennsylvania in August 2020, I wasn't scared. Yes, I was in pain from seeing so many of my people killed by police officers while people around the world lost their lives to COVID-19. I also struggled with the isolation of prolonged quarantines at the height of the pandemic. The circumstances of the pandemic made it impossible for me to meet my entire medical school class throughout my first year and postponed my white coat ceremony for over a year.

Despite the limited contact with my class, I found that prejudice still managed to seep through. At various points throughout the school year, I encountered colleagues who questioned whether my fellow black medical classmates and I had earned our spots at this prestigious medical school. We could be having a conversation about our medical school application cycle or our feelings about an impending exam, when a classmate would lay bare their views on the black medical students at Penn. They thought that our blackness, not our credentials, had given us access to this prestigious institution. Whenever I met these challenges, I kept my thoughts fixed on the incredible black women physicians who came before me. If they could do it, I could too.

As I trekked through those early days of medical school, I recognized that many students in my position didn't have the stories of these black women physicians to lighten their steps. Inundated with the dominant narrative that white men are the leaders of medicine, they didn't know how much black women had contributed to the field. If more black girls and women knew, maybe more would be inspired to pursue medicine. Maybe other underrepresented minorities in medicine would be inspired too.

Black women physicians' stories have gone untold for far too long, leaving gaping holes in American medical history, in women's history, and in black history. It's time to set the record straight.

AUTHOR'S NOTE

Throughout the book, I use the terms "black" and "African American" to describe the race and ethnicity of the women who are highlighted. Their varied use is both intentional and emotional. Both "black" and "African American" are terms that have been used to describe descendants of slavery in the United States. "Black" became a popular term to describe this community in the late 1960s and early 1970s.[2] Stokely Carmichael, who coined the term "Black Power," helped garner acceptance of this label within the community. Then, in 1988, Jesse Jackson suggested we replace "black" with "African American."[3] This switch to "African American" slowly gained popularity as a term to describe descendants of slavery in the US.

Now, "African American" is thought by many to be the more politically correct way to describe someone with my family history. "Black" has become an umbrella term to describe anyone in America with ancestors from Africa.

While black physicians were almost exclusively African American before the 1960s, our representation in the field has decreased markedly. Most black medical students are now recent African or Caribbean immigrants.[4] In my medical school class, there are about 160 students; 23 of them are black. While there are ten black women in my class, I am the only African American woman in the cohort. All ten of us can relate to the challenges of being black women in medicine, but there are unique barriers that come with being African American. In particular, the historical deprivation of educational and financial opportunities still makes it difficult for African Americans to access the medical profession today. This is a burden that my fellow black female classmates can't carry with me.

Sadly, this difference in experience has led to tensions in the larger black medical community. A few months before I started medical school, I reached out to older medical students for advice. At this stage, I was talking to students from multiple medical schools, and I hadn't decided which school I would commit to. I remember speaking to one black medical student from a prestigious school, a first-generation immigrant from an African country. He was trying to shake my fears about the demands of medical school. "Us Africans are so hardworking. You'll be fine."

My heart stopped. I recognized his bias and feared what he would think of me when he knew the truth. "I'm not African. I'm African American."

"Oh! Well, you're a Rhodes scholar. You must have a similar work ethic." His words made me ache with sadness. Was he implying that if I were just an African American, not an African American Rhodes scholar, he would think I wasn't as hardworking as my black classmates who were recent African or Caribbean immigrants? Too many times, black people from other ethnic groups have told me that African Americans are lazy. When this stereotype was perpetuated in the black medical space, there were few people I could turn to.

As I was writing this book, I chose to highlight African American women in particular to challenge this false narrative that African Americans are lazy. We had to work hard and exhibit unwavering determination to break into medicine. The immense obstacles impeding our journeys required nothing less. But we still shared many experiences with other black women physicians, and I hope that connection comes through too. These stories are meant to highlight the incredible achievements of the physicians who led the way, to inspire all people who have had to overcome discrimination along their journeys—and at the same time, I hope African American women, in particular, will recognize themselves in this book.

There are no invented quotes in this book. All scenes and dialogue are drawn either directly from oral history accounts, interviews I conducted, other primary resources, or a recounting of my own firsthand experience.

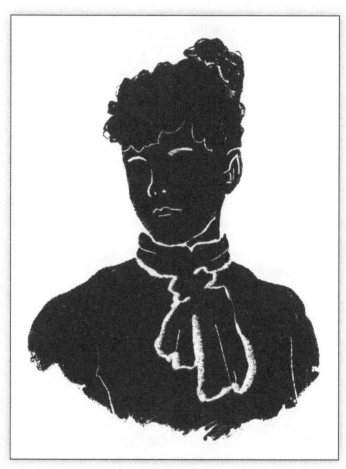

No images that can be verified
as Dr. Rebecca Lee Crumpler exist.

WITH DETERMINATION
AND FEARLESSNESS

Rebecca Lee Crumpler, born Rebecca Davis, became the first African American woman to earn a medical degree in the United States of America only fourteen months after President Abraham Lincoln signed the Emancipation Proclamation.

Rebecca was born free on February 8, 1831, in Christiana, Delaware, to Matilda Webber and Absolum Davis. During this time, the medical establishment was quite different from what it is today. In 1800, most American physicians were trained as apprentices of practicing physicians. The only American medical schools that offered lectures to augment the clinical apprenticeships were the University of Pennsylvania, Harvard University, and Dartmouth College. Some wealthy men would acquire their medical educations abroad, primarily in Edinburgh, Scotland. In 1800, approximately one hundred Edinburgh-trained physicians, plus the graduates from the three American institutions, constituted a medical elite.[1] This group, combined with those who trained as apprentices, were described as the "regular physicians," or allopaths. This medical sect competed with two others: the homeopaths and the eclectics. They all had different approaches to treating patients, and they all sought to portray their form of medicine as the most logical and effective.

Rebecca was raised in Pennsylvania by her aunt, who was likely an herbalist. As a child, Rebecca would see sick people file into her home. They arrived with a sense of urgency and distress. Many of them seemed to leave with newfound hope and relief after visiting her aunt. Seeing the impact her aunt was making in her community sparked a passion inside of Rebecca. She decided that she, too, wanted to be a healer when she grew up. Somehow (and records are absent here) she completed her studies at the prestigious West Newton English and Classical School in Newton, Massachusetts, just miles outside of Boston, and then moved to nearby Charlestown, Massachusetts, in 1852, to work as a nurse.[2]

What made Rebecca pursue work as a nurse instead of as a doctor? While the unique work experience of being a nurse might have been more appealing than that of being a doctor, access to medical training likely played a role in her decision. Rebecca was not the first African American woman in history to want to become a physician. She was not even the first African American woman who had the skills necessary to be a great physician. Prior to the 1860s, immense social and structural barriers prevented countless aspiring African American women physicians from achieving their dreams. Rebecca was the first to break this near-impenetrable blockade. At the time, physicians were almost exclusively white men. African American men and white women were just starting to gain access to the field. The experiences of these early physicians show some of the impediments that halted many African American women in their medical journeys. These impediments made Rebecca's path so difficult, and so remarkable.

The first person to break the color barrier in medicine was James McCune Smith. Born a slave in 1813, James had more opportunities than many other slaves. His owner allowed him to attend the New York African Free School No. 2, a school that taught black boys. In 1827, a year before he graduated, he gained his freedom through the Emancipation Act of the State of New York. Suddenly, the possibilities for James's future were endless. He decided he wanted to become a physician. He worked as a blacksmith to support himself while studying Latin and Greek, two languages that medical schools required their students to be fluent in.

Following these rigorous studies, James applied to Columbia College and Geneva, two medical schools in New York. The schools' decisions: denied on account of his race. James was refused an American medical education, but he did not give up on his goal. He applied to the University of Glasgow, a prestigious college in Scotland, and was admitted.

Excited about James's accomplishment, black professionals in his community raised enough money to send him to this school in 1832.

Dr. McCune Smith returned to the US from Scotland in 1837 with his BA, MA, and MD degrees from the University of Glasgow. He had found a way to navigate higher education in a country he had never been to, attaining three degrees in five years. This was an incredible feat that required a sharp mind and diligence. Unfortunately, there was also an unspoken requirement. While this school was more open to educating black men than most universities in the world, it refused to teach women, regardless of their ethnicities. It wasn't until 1892 that women were finally allowed to matriculate into any university in Scotland. The University of Glasgow didn't become completely coed until the 1930s, and even then women were segregated in separate learning quarters, through to the 1950s.[3] These Scottish schools could stomach a man with a different skin color, but a woman was just too much to bear.

While Dr. McCune Smith was completing his medical training in Scotland, anti-abolitionist sentiment was brewing in New York. In July 1834, white Americans who feared even baby steps toward racial equality joined forces to incite a three-day riot in New York City. It has been described as the worst riot in antebellum America.[4] Mobs targeted dozens of black homes and set them aflame. They also targeted institutions that sought to bring African Americans out of poverty and prepare them for the job market. Dr. McCune Smith's New York African Free School was one of the black institutions burned down.

Were these white people angered that the school helped a black person prepare for medical school? Or was it the school's general aim to teach black boys how to read and write that incited their violence? Regardless of the specific motivations, this terrorist attack sent fear through the free black community in antebellum America. Like the severe punishment slaves endured when they tried to claim their freedom, this act of violence was a warning for any other black person who strove to have a successful career in America. If they made any advances in society, that black person, along with their beloved community, would experience great loss. Many black and white Americans advocating for a more equal society became more hesitant in their push for change. The backlash likely caused some black children interested in medicine to give up their dream. Rebecca was only three years old at the time. As a consequence, from the moment that she was old enough to interpret social dynamics in her environment, she probably understood that aiming too high in society, as a black American, could result in tragedy.

Although Dr. McCune Smith returned to a community whose members had been made to fear their own advancement, he bravely held on to his newfound position within medicine. He opened a medical practice and the country's first black-owned pharmacy, at 55 West Broadway in New York City. He attracted black and white patients due to his strong reputation. Even racist white doctors respected his expertise, as evidenced by his medical publications.[5] He practiced medicine for about twenty-five years. Dr. McCune Smith's clinical practice was the first foothold in medicine for black Americans. The next necessary step to make medical careers accessible for the black community was to allow them to train in US schools.

In the 1830s, medicine was in the process of professionalizing. There was no licensing system. Anyone could practice as a physician. As a result, systematic discrimination occurred primarily around admission to medical school. Fifteen years passed between Dr. McCune Smith's rejection from American medical schools and the graduation of the first African American from an American medical school. All women were still being excluded from medical training programs in the US.

David Jones Peck was born free in 1826 or 1827 in Carlisle, Pennsylvania, to John C. and Sarah ("Sally") Peck, two freed black people who worked to help other black Americans gain their freedom and attain educations. John Peck was one of the primary financial supporters of the Underground Railroad in Pennsylvania.[6] While Pennsylvania became the first of the colonies to pass an abolition law in 1780, white Philadelphians had slaves throughout David's time at Rush Medical College in Chicago, which was from 1846 to 1847. His parents' support was essential as he withstood the emotional toll of having classmates who had the ability to own one of his family members as their slave.

Some of his medical school classmates likely held the view that African Americans were property, not people, prompting them to object to David's presence in the class. While the faculty believed that David was qualified to join the medical school, the president of the college allowed the white male students to decide if David could join their class. In a time when a large portion of American society thought that a black American's main purpose in life was to serve and submit to white men, qualifications didn't matter. All that mattered was the color of one's skin.

The white male medical students were left alone in a classroom to discuss the issue. With so many white men having roamed the halls before them, they felt assured of their right to hold space in the class. But what about "the darkey," as one of David's classmates referred to him? Could he really fit in with them? Would they accept someone who could've been their slave to instead be their medical school classmate? There was fierce debate. In the end, there were just enough willing to vote for David's continued presence at the school. If a few more bigoted white men had been admitted that year, David might not have been allowed to become a doctor. Instead, he was permitted to matriculate. He graduated from Rush in the spring of 1847.

If Rebecca had been in David's place, would the same group of white men have voted in her favor? Because no woman had been allowed to study in a medical school in the US, or anywhere in the world, up to this point, they almost certainly would've voted to remove her from the class. The school's faculty probably wouldn't have advocated for her based on her credentials. There was still a certain look required to make it in medicine. A woman, white or black, didn't fit the bill.

This demand for all doctors to be men didn't start to change until 1849, when Elizabeth Blackwell earned her medical degree from Geneva Medical College in New York. Born in 1821 in Bristol, England, to a middle-class family, Elizabeth had more professional connections than a black woman like Rebecca Davis. When she decided to pursue medicine, following her move to the United States, she reached out to physicians whom she knew for advice. The path to medicine is usually difficult, regardless of the aspiring physician's identity. It is extremely long, with many hidden costs and hurdles. Having a physician-mentor can make a big difference in navigating this journey. The remarkable advantage of having such support explains why the vast majority of medical students today have either parents or family friends who are physicians.[7] Elizabeth had this support system. But in an era when most white Americans were against the true equality of the races and almost every physician was white, it was very difficult for a black woman like Rebecca to find a physician-mentor who would guide her along her journey.

Unfortunately, many of the physicians in Elizabeth's network tried to discourage her pursuit of a medical career. She was a woman; it wasn't practical for her to go into medicine. The conditions were too harsh and the exposed bodies too vulgar. The fact that she would even consider such a profession raised concerns in some physicians: if she could envision herself as a doctor, was she really a lady? These men's reactions showed Elizabeth that she would be fighting against the suffocating social norms that tried to force women into a peripheral realm of society, limiting what they were capable of achieving in their lives. If Elizabeth was successful, she could loosen the corset on women's lives and allow them to move freely toward a world filled with possibilities.

After talking to multiple physicians, Elizabeth finally found someone who was willing to help. He provided her with a list of US medical schools. This glimmer of support made all the difference. She began by applying to four medical schools in Philadelphia, the epicenter of American medicine in the 1840s. After investing her precious time and money to attend interviews at these schools, she was met with cutting laughter.[8] The male physicians found it hilarious that a woman would even attempt to enter the medical field. Who did Elizabeth think she was?

She was a woman who was not easily deterred. Even after being rejected from school after school, she stood firm in her ambitions. She was unwilling to concede. One doctor was impressed by her determination. Trying to be helpful, he outlined steps other women had taken in their attempts to acquire medical training: Cut your hair. Trade your dress for pants. Hide a side of yourself that you've been taught to accentuate your whole life. This is a men's club. To be accepted in any capacity, you must look the part.[9] He told her she might find some success if she dressed as a man and attended medical lectures in Paris. Because she wasn't born a male, she wouldn't be allowed to earn a medical degree, but her disguise would at least grant her access to medical knowledge.

Elizabeth refused. She recognized her purpose as paving the way for women in medicine. To do this, she needed to remove the rocks in the road that impeded her medical journey, and those of numerous other women. This required her to face male intolerance and find a way into medicine while remaining easily identifiable as a woman. While the physicians detested her womanhood, they likely found some solace in her whiteness. The image of what a doctor should look like wouldn't be shattered irrevocably.

Elizabeth continued her turbulent path with more applications. The New York College of Physicians and Surgeons. Jefferson Medical College. Yale School of Medicine. University of Vermont College of Medicine. And many more. Rejection, rejection, rejection. Still, she pressed on. Elizabeth's third round of applications encompassed submissions to twelve smaller medical schools. The response was overwhelming denial. These schools refused to allow a woman to join their ranks, even after she had gained support from established physicians.

One medical school was different. The dean of Geneva Medical College, Dr. Charles Lee, wanted to be respectful of the doctor who had recommended Elizabeth. Instead of rejecting Elizabeth outright, he repeated with her the circumstances that Dr. David Jones Peck had endured after he gained admission to his medical school. Dr. Lee left it to a vote. The white men who would be Elizabeth's classmates had the power to decide her fate. But the dean didn't want a woman at his medical school, so he tried to stack the odds in his favor. Of the 150 men who composed the medical school body, only one had to say "no" for Elizabeth to be rejected.[10] But these white male students responded in a fashion similar to that of some physicians who had interviewed Elizabeth. When they found out that a woman was trying to enter their ranks, they were sent into fits of laughter.[11] How could a woman think that she could become a physician? In the end, these men were too entertained by the comic notion of a lady doctor to let the moment pass. Elizabeth's soon-to-be classmates voted to admit her to the school in October 1847, months after Dr. David Jones Peck earned his medical degree. To her classmates, the vote to accept Elizabeth was simply a hilarious joke. To Elizabeth and the white women who came after her, it was the foothold they needed to finally pierce the medical world. Soon after Dr. Elizabeth Blackwell graduated from medical school in 1849, new colleges of medicine explicitly and exclusively for women began to open, which allowed hundreds of white women to join the medical profession.

D espite these advances for white women and black men, progress was still stalled for black women. The unique obstacles of being black, and those of being a woman, were multiplied for people with both identities, slowing black women's entry to the medical field. Rebecca Davis heard about, and possibly even encountered, this shifting demographic of physicians while she worked as a nurse. She also developed physician-mentors who pointed her to more progressive institutions. Howard University College of Medicine, the first historically black American medical school, didn't open until 1868. Therefore, Rebecca's best chance of being trained as a physician was through one of the new crop of women's medical colleges. When she ambitiously applied to medical school in 1860, there were only 300 women out of 54,543 physicians in the US. None of those women were black.[12]

Rebecca was accepted at the New England Female Medical College in 1860. She was the school's only black student in its twenty-five-year history.[13] In this space that supported women, the challenges of being black in America had not even been broached. Rebecca slogged through a demanding medical school curriculum alongside her white classmates with a constant threat hanging over her head. A white person could inflict violence upon her or her community for evading slavery and taking strides toward prosperity. Violent opposition to abolition had persisted in the North for decades. The multiday riot in New York that demolished Dr. McCune Smith's community in 1834 had not been the first, nor was it the last. Proslavery violence occurred in Boston during Rebecca's childhood and early adulthood. Hate crimes were a response to the strong abolitionist presence in the city.

When Abraham Lincoln was elected president of the United States in November 1860, during Rebecca's first year of medical school, the violence in Boston intensified. While Lincoln believed that white southerners had the right to enslave other people in perpetuity, he was against the expansion of slavery to the West.[14] This outraged many white Americans. Lincoln's position threatened their pocketbooks and their dominance within society. It prompted eleven southern states to secede and form the Confederacy between his election and his inauguration, a period referred to as the Secession Winter of 1860 and 1861.

Although Lincoln spoke only about halting the expansion of slavery, abolitionists saw this as their opportunity to end slavery altogether. They advocated for this change through public demonstrations and political lobbying. On a chilly December day in 1860, Boston abolitionists held a public meeting at Tremont Temple to strategize on how to eradicate American slavery. Frederick Douglass was among many prominent leaders of the abolitionist movement who spoke. White Bostonians who supported slavery caught wind of this meeting and mobilized. They filled the lecture hall, outnumbering the abolitionists. When Douglass tried to deliver his speech, angry white men pulled him off the platform by his gray-streaked curly hair. Immediately, the hall broke out in violence. The police were present and watched this scene. Eventually, they removed the abolitionists from the hall, allowing the white anti-abolitionists to control the event. While this did subdue the crowd, the abolitionists were furious that the white Bostonians who started the violence, and who were in support of slavery, had upended their event with the help of the police.

After the leaders of the event lumbered away from Tremont Temple, they regrouped to discuss a way to resume their meeting that evening. They decided on the African Meeting House on Joy Street, only two miles from Rebecca's medical school. When the anti-abolitionists found out about their plans, they recruited even more white men to intimidate the group holding the event. The police changed their tactics, allowing the abolitionists to speak, while keeping the slavery supporters outside. The street filled with thousands of angry white men, many of whom by their dress appeared to have come from well-paid jobs. They tensely waited to respond to the abolitionists.

Once the meeting ended, the police force abandoned the scene, while the irate crowd remained. These white men had brought axes, clubs, and stones to the meeting, and they leveled them at the black Bostonians exiting the African Meeting House. A few rioters even used guns. Cracked bones. Splattered blood. Cries of agony. This was the impact the well-off white men had on a black community that just wanted freedom for their brethren. Some of the black people were brought to the brink of death.[15]

Not yet satisfied with the torment they had inflicted on the abolitionists in the meeting, the white mob took to nearby black neighborhoods, shattering windows and ripping furniture apart. They wanted to do what they could to destroy the few comforts these freed black families had found in the more progressive North. The terrorists took to the trolley cars traveling on Cambridge Street near the north slope of Beacon Hill. They dragged the black passengers off the trolley and beat them senseless.

By this point, the Boston police had been notified of the violence in the black neighborhoods. Large groups of police officers, all white, stalked the streets as the heinous assault occurred. But they did nothing to stop the attack. They must not have been concerned by the severe harm their white brothers were inflicting on this black community. Maybe they applauded their efforts. Maybe they would've joined the crowd with their own clubs if they hadn't been on duty. The only person they arrested was a black boy who tried to defend himself after white assailants broke into and destroyed his home.[16] Apparently, it was legal for a white man to ransack a black family's home. If a black man did this to a white family's home in the 1800s, he might be punished by hanging. But the rules were different for white men. Incidents of white anti-abolitionists attacking black Bostonians increased dramatically following this tragic event.

It is unclear if Rebecca or someone close to her was a victim of the assaults. Since the attacks occurred only two miles away from her school, it's very possible that she was personally impacted by the violence. But even if Rebecca avoided being physically harmed, fear surely struck her heart. She decided to take time off from medical school and relocate to Richmond, Virginia, for a while.[17] The anti-abolitionists in Boston were too dangerous for her to remain there.

Rebecca's medical school did not care that her life was in danger when the Civil War erupted. It stripped her of the scholarship that had made it possible for her to attend. But her foot was already in the door. Refusing to let this deeply rooted dream slip away, she fervently sought other funding. She was eventually awarded the Wade Scholarship, established by abolitionist Benjamin Wade.[18] Once she returned to school, she had to keep her nose in her books. She couldn't worry about what would happen if the Confederacy won the Civil War. She couldn't entertain the possibility of slavery returning to the North. She was expected to perform on par with her white classmates, so that's what she did.

When Lincoln issued the Emancipation Proclamation on January 1, 1863, Rebecca must have been elated. For the final fourteen months of her medical education, she could breathe more easily. She wouldn't be sold into slavery. And the African Americans enslaved in the South could finally claim their freedom. Dr. Rebecca Lee Davis triumphantly graduated from medical school in 1864. This was twenty-seven years after black men—and fifteen years after white women—had been allowed to become physicians.

Once Dr. Davis entered the medical sphere, she faced immense resistance and skepticism. She needed a protective shield to weather the harsh conditions of a largely racist and sexist medical community. For her, this armor would be gleaned from her work caring for others in need. After she graduated from medical school, she married Arthur Crumpler and changed her name to Dr. Rebecca Lee Crumpler.[19] Arthur understood her need to support disenfranchised people, and he supported her career. Together, they moved to Richmond to serve with the Freedmen's Bureau, a government-sanctioned group meant to help the four million newly freed African Americans transition into society.[20] Many of these people had been deprived of proper healthcare all their lives.

While the other healthcare providers claimed to care about the plight of African Americans, they did not wish for a just society. Their treatment of Dr. Crumpler proved that they didn't want African Americans, or at least not African American women, as their medical colleagues. Administrators tried to prevent her from admitting patients, and pharmacists refused to fill her prescriptions.[21] They could not believe that a black woman was capable of being a competent physician. Some of the male physicians jeered: "The MD behind her name stands for nothing more than 'Mule Driver.'"[22] While Dr. Crumpler likely felt disheartened by her colleagues' demeaning behavior, caring for the African American community kept her going. She remembered the experience as "a proper field for real missionary work, and one that would present ample opportunities to become acquainted with the diseases of women and children. During my stay there nearly every hour was improved in that sphere of labor."[23]

In 1869, Dr. Crumpler and her husband moved back to Boston after spending about five years in Virginia. They bought a home on Joy Street in Beacon Hill, the very same black neighborhood that had been destroyed by angry white anti-abolitionists during her first year of medical school. Many of her neighbors likely still had the scars from that horrid day. Dr. Crumpler used her home as her medical office. Members of the community filed in seeking relief for their ailments. She mainly served black women and children, as she had in Virginia. It didn't matter if they had the funds to pay for their visit. She would treat them regardless.[24]

During the decade or so that she maintained this private practice, her medical sect, allopathic medicine, was changing drastically. The groundwork for this change was laid while she was still practicing as a nurse. In 1855, German physician Rudolf Virchow proposed that cells came from preexisting cells. This differed from the prevailing view, that new cells arose from a fluid called blastema. Imbalance of blastema was thought to cause disease. Virchow leveraged his opposing theory to develop the field of cellular pathology: the study of disease at the cellular level.[25] In 1861, French chemist Louis Pasteur added on to this reductionist approach to medicine.[26] He proposed the germ theory, that the invasion of microorganisms into the body can cause disease.[27] In 1876, German physician Robert Koch applied Pasteur's germ theory to investigate the causative agent of the deadly anthrax disease. He found the bacterium *Bacillus anthracis* to be that agent. This was the first time someone had scientifically proven that a specific microorganism caused a specific disease.[28] He later discovered the causative agents of a few other deadly infectious diseases, including tuberculosis and cholera.[29] The baton of innovation was passed back to Pasteur in 1879, when he serendipitously immunized chickens against cholera. He accomplished this by inoculating the chickens with a live-attenuated version of *Vibrio cholerae*, the bacterium that causes cholera. He used this technique to develop vaccines against anthrax and rabies.[30]

As these European discoveries gained acceptance, they profoundly influenced American medical practice. In the 1870s, allopathic doctors' use of bleeding and calomel, a popular purgative, decreased drastically.[31] Instead, with insight from scientific experiments, they started to use specific therapies for specific diseases. This new therapeutic strategy was easier to tolerate and seemed more effective than the broad and drastic measures that doctors had used traditionally. The shift toward scientific medicine boosted the public's confidence in allopathic medicine.[32] It's likely that Dr. Crumpler applied these innovations to her medical practice.

In 1880, Dr. Crumpler and her husband moved to Hyde Park, another neighborhood in Boston. There are no records to show whether she continued her medical practice in the new community. But even if she wasn't seeing patients on a regular basis, she continued working to improve the health of her community. When she was fifty-two years old, she published *A Book of Medical Discourses: In Two Parts*, which leveraged her more than twenty years of clinical experience, both as a nurse and a doctor, providing medical advice to women on topics such as washing and dressing a newborn, breastfeeding, maintaining proper nutrition, managing diphtheria and measles, and treating burns.[33] The book was especially helpful for black women who couldn't find a doctor that they could afford. It equipped them with the knowledge to care for themselves. The work further marked her as a pioneer; it is the only known medical book written by a nineteenth-century African American woman.[34] Dr. Crumpler passed away twelve years later, on March 9, 1895.

D id Dr. Crumpler ever know that she was the first black woman physician in the country? Or that she was the only black woman to publish a medical book in America in the nineteenth century? She wasn't celebrated for breaking these barriers, the way Dr. McCune Smith or Dr. Blackwell were. There were no news articles about her that were published while she was alive. No photographs were taken to cement her legacy. There is an image that accompanies Dr. Crumpler's name in internet searches, but that image is not of Dr. Crumpler—it's Mary Eliza Mahoney, the first African American to become a professionally trained nurse in the United States.

I had studied Mary's photo in countless articles describing Dr. Crumpler's medical journey. Mary's picture brought Dr. Crumpler's story to life in my mind. When I stumbled upon an article that revealed that this picture was actually of a different person, I was shocked. I searched Mary Mahoney's image to double check. Sure enough, the same woman stared back at me. The cognitive dissonance sent a flash of emotion through my body. Is this how little they thought of us black women? That it was unfathomable that we could've become physicians in the nineteenth century? At best, we became nurses. I couldn't point to just sexism or racism. It was sexist because women in the medical sphere were oftentimes assumed to be nurses instead of doctors. It was racist because nineteenth-century white women physicians had been widely recognized, while nineteenth-century black women physicians were ignored. Maybe it was our blackness juxtaposed against our womanliness. As the antithesis of the poster child for medicine—a white male doctor—the image of black women as physicians must've been too preposterous to imagine.

I felt even worse when I found out that historians didn't always recognize Dr. Rebecca Crumpler as the first black woman physician.

Without sources like newspaper clippings, the introduction of *A Book of Medical Discourses: In Two Parts* is one of the only primary sources in existence that details Dr. Crumpler's life. For a while, historians didn't realize that Dr. Crumpler made this medical milestone. They thought Dr. Rebecca J. Cole, the second black woman physician, was actually the first.[35] I couldn't believe that historians had made this mistake. But even if no one thought her work was important enough to document at the time, Dr. Crumpler's achievements are too powerful for her to remain invisible.

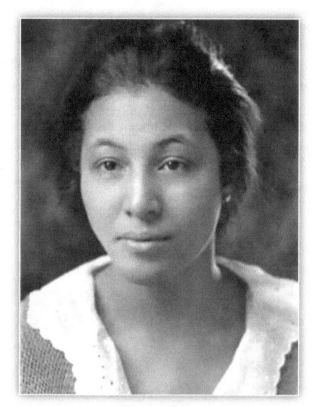

Dr. May Chinn

DOING SURGERY IN THE BEDROOM

The nineteenth century passed with a whisper of hope. It seemed like the door that Dr. Rebecca Lee Crumpler had cracked open was gradually widening. More black women joined the medical profession. In 1890, thirty-six years after Dr. Crumpler earned her medical degree, there were 115 black women physicians in the US. The steady rise continued through to 1900, when 160 black women were in the profession.[1] But this optimism about progress must be paired with perspective. How did a black woman's access to the medical profession at the turn of the twentieth century compare to that of her counterparts?

In that same year that black women physicians reached 160, there were approximately 88,000 white male physicians, 3,500 white female physicians, and 1,600 black male physicians.[2] According to the census of 1901, there were almost 67 million white Americans and 9 million black Americans, both split approximately evenly between men and women.[3] Based on this data, 1 out of every 375 white men was a physician. One out of every 2,800 black men was a physician. One out of every 9,430 white women was a physician. And 1 out of every 28,125 black women was a physician. Black women were still drastically underrepresented.

When allopathic physicians considered how their medical community was developing at the turn of the twentieth century, many were concerned.[4] Their opinions on the demographic shift varied. But a large portion believed that the total number of US physicians was too high. This was due to the significant increase in medical schools. Between 1800 and 1900, approximately four hundred medical schools were founded.[5] This heightened competition in the medical workforce, both within the allopathic sect and between the other medical sects. As a result, each individual physician had fewer patients and a lower income.

Allopathic physicians had tried, and failed, to reduce this competition in the nineteenth century. But as science-based therapies became more central to the doctors' practice, eliminating the competition became more feasible. In the nineteenth century, medical faculties relied on student fees for their incomes. The more students they had, the more money they made. This fueled the boom in medical trainees. But once students completed their training, they entered the workforce. With so many physicians, it was difficult for an individual physician to make as much money as they wanted. As a result, the practicing physicians wanted fewer students entering the medical pipeline.

The medical faculty members and practicing physicians were on opposing sides of this issue until science-based research made new clinical methods possible. The introduction of anesthesia and antiseptics in the mid to late nineteenth century eliminated intense pain and deadly infections from the typical surgical experience. Physicians could charge more for these specialized surgeries. This became a major source of income for many medical faculty members. As a result, they became invested in promoting "medical science." These faculty members raised the standards of their medical schools to ensure that they remained abreast of the new scientific approach to medicine, which resulted in fewer medical school admissions every year. Just what the medical practitioners wanted.

At the turn of the twentieth century, the new medical scientists joined forces with elite medical practitioners. Together, they took control of the American Medical Association (AMA). They reshaped this national institution, which was founded in 1847, into "the profession's instrument of political action."[6] They set standards that all medical schools were expected to adhere to. They were to admit students with at least four years of high school education. With only 15 percent of high school age Americans enrolled in high school at the time, this requirement favored middle- and upper-class white men for medical school admissions.[7]

In addition, the medical schools were to provide four years of education, not short one-year courses that were popular in the nineteenth century. The schools also needed adequate laboratory and clinical teaching facilities, as well as a highly trained laboratory and clinical faculty. Finally, the medical students were to pass an exam before they could attain their state license. Medical education reformers in the AMA joined the state medical licensing boards to push their agenda.[8] Reformers pushed for local laws that barred students from taking medical licensing exams if the students attended a medical school that didn't meet these standards, driving many students to AMA-approved medical schools. This, and multiple other medical education reform efforts, caused forty-four medical schools to close or merge between 1904 and 1909.[9]

But reformers weren't satisfied with these results. They enlisted the Carnegie Foundation for the Advancement of Teaching, which was founded in 1905, to create a uniform higher education system to expand reform efforts. Once the foundation was convinced these reforms would align with its own values, it agreed to fund a survey of medical schools throughout the US and Canada. At the suggestion of Rockefeller Institute director Dr. Simon Flexner, the Carnegie Foundation invited Simon's brother Abraham Flexner to lead the study.[10] Abraham Flexner was a trained educator and former high school teacher, but he had no experience with the medical education system. He didn't have a job when he received the offer from the Carnegie Foundation. Despite his limited knowledge of the field, he happily accepted.

Following his tour of medical schools, Abraham Flexner published what is now known as the Flexner Report of 1910. The report's recommendations closely echoed those of the reformers leading the AMA. Flexner advocated for improved facilities and better, scientifically trained faculties. Johns Hopkins, his alma mater, was the standard he encouraged all medical schools to aspire to. Johns Hopkins University School of Medicine was modeled after the German medical education system, which used evidence from biomedical research to shape their therapeutic interventions. Given the influence that German scientists and physicians were having on the development of biomedicine, this high standard pushed American medical schools to modernize. It helped our medical education system gain the eminence it enjoys to this day.

However, Flexner criticized medical schools for training too many doctors. He advised schools to require all incoming students to have at least two years of college education. With only 5 percent of college age Americans in college at the time, this steered medical schools even further to draw incoming students primarily from the elite classes, now welcoming only those with a high school diploma and some college education.[11] Purging the physician workforce of poor and working-class people is something that the reformers wanted. Flexner's recommendations helped them achieve it.

The report also introduced new barriers for black Americans interested in medicine, particularly impacting black women. The report suggested that male and female medical students should be trained together but perpetuated the segregation of black students from their white counterparts. The New England Female Medical College, Dr. Crumpler's alma mater, and Woman's Medical College of Pennsylvania, Dr. Cole's alma mater, were among a handful of women's medical colleges founded in the nineteenth century. They played a central role in training women from all backgrounds. Following the Flexner Report, the three women's medical colleges that had survived into the twentieth century were forced to merge with white male-dominated medical schools. Because racial segregation was maintained, the mergers meant fewer opportunities for black women to be trained in medicine. The limited spots designated for women at the white male-dominated schools would be given almost exclusively to white women.

Aligned with the racist views of the time, Flexner argued that black physicians should treat only black patients. And, as he wrote in his report, "the fewer, the better."[12] At least fourteen black medical schools or departments had been founded in the late nineteenth century.[13] Only seven survived to the early twentieth century. After Flexner's report, the number was slashed to two: Howard University College of Medicine and Meharry Medical College.[14] The medical reformers in the AMA were happy with this change. There would be fewer black physicians to threaten the racial hierarchy or to compete with white physicians in the job market. In 1918, the AMA pushed for the closure of Meharry. But the Carnegie Foundation stepped in and provided financial support for the school.[15] Howard and Meharry became the primary avenues for black Americans to acquire medical training. At this time, it was a popular view that men should predominate within the medical profession. Thus, these two medical schools likely favored admission of black men in the early twentieth century, further stifling opportunities for black women.

The adoption of Flexner's suggestions by medical schools around the country immediately halted the progress of black women in medicine. The wide-reaching and long-lasting impediments still exist today. By 1920, the number of black women physicians had toppled to sixty-five, less than half the number in 1900.[16] Strikingly, the changes implemented due to this report became a persistent blockade to African Americans' access to medicine. Almost one hundred years after the report was published, the percentage of black physicians was actually lower than it had been right before the implementation of Flexner's recommendations. In 1910, 2.5 percent of all physicians were black; by 2006, that number had dropped to 2.2 percent.[17] How did this changing climate impact African American women who sought to enter medicine, when there were only sixty-five in the field? Dr. May Chinn's story gives us a clue of the broader experience of black women entering medicine at this time.

On a crisp spring day in 1896, May Chinn was born in Great Barrington, Massachusetts. Neither her mother, Lulu Ann, nor her father, William Lafayette Chinn, had a college education. They represented the vast majority of African Americans at the time, who were not allowed to attain an education. May's father had been born into slavery. He seized his freedom at eleven years old when he bravely ran away from the Chinn plantation in Virginia. He never spoke about his painful experiences as a slave. He focused on the pride he felt from outwitting his captors with his escape.

May's mother, Lulu, was twenty-four years younger than May's father. She was born free in 1876 but worked as a servant for a wealthy white family who moved from Virginia to Massachusetts. Lulu was determined to lead her daughter down a different path. She believed that a strong education would give May an easier life. But the *Plessy v. Ferguson* Supreme Court case was decided a month after May was born. The ruling codified racial segregation laws in numerous societal institutions, including the education system. This left May to be taught at all-black schools that were deprived of educational resources and adequate government funding.

Despite these challenges, Lulu did what she could to support her child. She worked as a live-in cook for Charles Tiffany, the founder of Tiffany & Co. jewelers, and his family. She earned an extremely modest income. William's job prospects were even worse. Like many African American men in the early 1900s, he was unable to acquire a skilled job due to racial discrimination.[18] His only options were low-paying jobs, like mail carrier. His employment status was unstable, his income sparse. The heavy burden of providing for the family lay on Lulu with her meager income. Still, she saved every penny that she could for May's education. Eventually, she saved up enough money to send May to the Bordentown Manual Training and Industrial School, a New Jersey boarding school for African Americans.

While May was at boarding school, she fell ill. Her forehead was hot to the touch. Her legs and arms swelled in pain. She had osteomyelitis, a bone infection, and had to undergo an extensive surgery, which required a long period in recovery. This prevented May from fulfilling her responsibilities at school. She was taken out of school and brought to live with her mother at the Tiffany family's Irvington estate, in upstate New York.

Life with the Tiffanys exposed May to a whole new world: the bright lights of New York City, the vibrant colors of the circus, exquisite musical arrangements at Walter Damrosch concerts. May accompanied the Tiffany children on many of their adventures. She even sat in on their homeschool lessons on topics like French and German.[19] This rich cultural exposure planted in May seeds of interest in areas such as music, which bloomed later in her life.

Maybe wealthy families like the Tiffanys took pity on their black domestic workers' children. The children weren't a direct threat to the family's superior position in society. Even if the children were educated, they couldn't compete with the white children for job opportunities when they grew up. As a result, some black children in the early twentieth century gained secondhand exposure to educational enrichment activities from their mothers' wealthy employers.[20]

Not long after May moved to the Irvington estate, Charles Tiffany died, and the estate was broken up. May and her mother moved back in with May's father, in Lower Manhattan. From that point on, the family constantly hopped from one neighborhood to another. At one point they lived at Columbus Circle, right across from the lush Central Park. After May completed grammar school, the family uprooted again and moved to the Bronx.

It wasn't until May was much older that she realized their constant moving was motivated by her mother's attempts to get her into the best schools possible. When May was a teenager, some schools had started to desegregate. Lulu saw this as an opportunity to get her baby in a school with better resources. First, she enrolled May in Washington Irving High School, a good, predominantly black high school in Manhattan. But when the highly regarded Morris High School in the Bronx desegregated, Lulu jumped at the opportunity to enroll her daughter. When Lulu realized that Morris High was too far of a commute from their Manhattan residence, she promptly moved her family closer to the school.

May didn't always appreciate the sacrifices her mother made for her. She didn't understand the long-term implications of attending a well-resourced high school. Like many teenagers, she was just living in the moment. May followed her mother's plan during freshman and sophomore year of high school. But when she became a junior, things changed. May felt cheated by her eleventh-grade Latin teacher, who gave her a lower grade than she felt she deserved. This may have been due to racism. Or the teacher may have graded her fairly. Regardless of what caused it, the low Latin grade haunted her. May was used to performing well in school.

If this wasn't bad enough, her spirits were further dampened by a love turned sour. She was charmed by an older, Greek man with olive-colored skin. He was a vegetable store owner, a widower with three children. Things started off light and fun. May would go to the store after school to see him and play with his children. She was moved by her emotions for him, but she didn't realize his intentions.

Being a widower, the man wanted a woman to complete his family. Someone to take care of his kids. May was only sixteen years old, but the man decided May could fill this motherly role. With little warning, he asked May to be his wife and the mother to his children. May was completely shocked. She wasn't ready to be a mother. She was still figuring out who she was. So, she bravely turned down the proposal. But her decision had consequences.

First, turning down the man's proposal meant ending her romance with him. This left her heartbroken.[21] Even worse for May than this new feeling of grief, the decision fractured her relationship with her father. In a 1979 interview, despite her eighty-three years, May easily recalled this change. "My father just washed his hands completely of me. He hardly spoke with me."[22] Her father's denouncement left May completely distraught. This was the blow that finally broke her. May lost the drive to continue working hard in school. With only a year left of high school, she dropped out.

May was quickly plunged into the adult world. She needed a job to support herself, so she gravitated toward music. Throughout her childhood, she had attended piano lessons funded by her mother's scant income. May used this training to teach kindergarten-age children. The lessons ranged from traditional piano lessons to complex skits that the kids performed at the YMCA and at social events. This work gave her great joy. She didn't feel like she was missing out by not finishing high school.

Her mother, on the other hand, was grieved. She wanted more for her daughter. So she continued to push May to further her education. Through fervent networking, Lulu found out that May could still gain admission into college if she took an entrance exam. She begged May to take the test, and May hesitantly agreed. May assumed that she wouldn't do well. Instead, her potential shone through; she performed so well that she gained admission to the prestigious Teachers College at Columbia University. May was shocked by these results. They made her believe that maybe she could achieve more than she had previously thought possible. She started to see college as a great opportunity to challenge herself and further her knowledge.

When May's father found out about her college plans, his disapproval of her deepened. May explained: "His idea of a girl was that you got married and had children. See, he was a different generation. A girl that went to college became a queer woman. She didn't act like a woman. And he didn't want to be the father of a queer girl."[23] Because May didn't follow traditional gender roles, William refused to contribute to her education. He also avoided speaking to her for many years, even though they continued to live in the same house. Despite the tensions it brought to the family, Lulu and May remained committed to getting May through college.

In 1917, May began her studies at Columbia as a music major. Thanks to her high exam score, she had preemptively fulfilled almost all of her liberal arts requirements. She needed only one more prerequisite before she could fill her schedule exclusively with music classes, so she took two classes during her first semester of college. One was a music class with a German professor whose prejudiced thinking led him to use his position in the department to hinder May's advancement. May recognized this and sought a way to remedy the situation.

May's solace came from Dr. Jean Broadhurst, the professor of her sole non-music class, a biology course with a focus on bacteriology. Dr. Broadhurst was a white woman who did not allow any prejudice she had against African Americans to cloud her judgment of May. At the end of the semester, each student was assigned a topic for their final paper. Three days after turning hers in, May received a note from Dr. Broadhurst asking her to come by the office. When they met, Dr. Broadhurst explained that she wanted to meet May because she was impressed by her paper, especially since May was a music major. The professor spotted a blooming interest in science between the lines of May's writing. After discussing May's paper at length, Dr. Broadhurst said a handful of words that were like magic: "Well, if you ever make up your mind, if you decide to change your major, I think you have a future in science. So . . . you think about it."[24] This suggestion piqued May's interest, so she talked it over with her mom. The following year, with Lulu's approval, May switched her major from music to biological sciences.

As May progressed through college, the financial burden wore on her. She worked two jobs, as a piano accompanist of students majoring in music and as a lab technician in Dr. Broadhurst's lab. May fell in love with the process of learning. But she always feared that her next semester could be her last. She tried her best to enjoy each minute of learning while working as hard as she could to raise money for the next semester. And her mother was constantly fighting to earn enough to help May cover the cost of school.

Dr. Broadhurst helped by looking for new ways to make school more affordable for May. She encouraged May to take some clinical pathology classes at a postgraduate school in New York. These were less expensive classes that counted toward her degree requirements. They also made her a competitive job applicant in the burgeoning new field of clinical pathology. After May's junior year, she was hired as a clinical pathology technician at Flower Hospital on Fifth Avenue near the Rockefeller Institute. To manage her new day job and her coursework, she worked during the day and took her classes at night, as advised by Dr. Broadhurst.

At what point in May's schedule did she find time to study the material for the class? When did she have time for family obligations, never mind herself? I'm not sure how she was able to juggle these demanding commitments, especially since she finished her bachelor's degree far faster than students with fewer responsibilities completed theirs. As someone who was also on the premed track in college, I know it's a huge accomplishment to make it through this program in four years, especially while managing multiple jobs. I had friends who had jobs while school was in session. As they juggled the demands of school and work, many found themselves exhausted and extremely stressed. Some of them became so burnt out that they had to take time off to regain their energy or had to pivot toward a different career path. Only a few managed to hold multiple jobs, excel in their premedical classes, and maintain enough energy to overcome the unexpected hurdles along their medical journeys.

Music helped May stave off burnout in the midst of this demanding schedule. In addition to tutoring and accompanying students in Columbia's music department, May participated in small concerts at churches and at the YMCA. During one of these performances, a man approached her and said, "I understand that you're quite an accompanist. Would you mind accompanying me? Because it looks as though my accompanist is late."

May didn't have to turn around to see his face. She would recognize that voice anywhere. "Of course, Paul."[25] It was Paul Robeson. They went on to perform at many incredible music venues together. She accompanied Robeson and, sometimes, did a full performance by herself too.

Paul Robeson was, of course, a famous African American bass baritone concert artist and a leader of the Harlem Renaissance. May's time in the Tiffany household had introduced her to musical professionals and developed in her an abiding passion for the arts. This led her to continue to prioritize music in the midst of her demanding premedical curriculum. Serendipitously, May's need to work while she studied introduced her to a flourishing community of influential black musicians, whom she kept up with throughout her life.

During the few nights that she did go out, she had experiences that some might call historic. A friend would tell May the place and time for a hangout. Directions would lead to a humble storefront in Harlem. She would enter to find her friends seated at a round table. A candle at the center of the table created a warm and intimate atmosphere. After exchanging pleasantries, people would begin sharing their work. There were various black artists who held the floor, including famous writers like Langston Hughes, Countee Cullen, Jean Toomer, and Claude McKay.[26] After sharing what they had written, they would wait to see how their friends around the table responded. Sometimes May, or someone else at the table, would make a suggestion. This was where some popular works from the Harlem Renaissance came alive.

All the while, May continued performing with Paul Robeson. Sometimes they would sing and play piano at Madam C. J. Walker's recitals. Walker was an African American woman best known for her black haircare products, which helped her climb from poverty to become America's first female self-made millionaire.[27] May's relationships with these other black leaders and influencers indicate how small, and possibly tight-knit, the more professionally successful African American community was in New York in the late nineteenth and early twentieth centuries.

But May didn't let these awe-inspiring nights distract her from her research. The faculty at Flower Hospital's associated medical school, which taught homeopathic medicine, took note of May's work in the clinical pathology lab. The faculty members were so impressed that they offered her a full scholarship for four years of study in medicine if she would agree to teach her classmates clinical pathology. This news likely filled May with excitement. She had experienced countless instances where people told her she couldn't thrive in higher education because she was a black woman. Yet these faculty members believed in her and were convinced that May would be such a great contributor to medicine and their medical school, that they were willing to invest in her education.

Unsure of how to navigate this new situation, May went to her trusted mentor, Dr. Broadhurst, for advice. She was over the moon that May was considering a career in medicine but suggested a tweak in May's plans. She encouraged May to pursue allopathic schools, which were incorporating more scientific research-informed therapies into their practice. By the 1920s, this medical sect had gained definitive favor in American society over homeopathy. (Allopathic medicine has maintained its dominance to this day. What many people refer to as Western medicine, or biomedicine, is the modern form of allopathic medicine.)

As someone with parents who hadn't even been to college, May needed an advisor who could help her maximize her professional potential. American medicine was changing rapidly as May matured. How could she know that homeopathy, which had been popular for a large portion of the 1800s, was losing its prominence in society? To May, a medical school was a medical school. She didn't realize that her choice of a particular institution could have long-term implications for her career.

May might not have understood Dr. Broadhurst's preference for an allopathic school, but her professor hadn't steered her wrong yet. Following Dr. Broadhurst's advice, May applied to two allopathic medical schools: Columbia University Vagelos College of Physicians and Surgeons and New York University School of Medicine. Both medical schools have maintained prominence in the medical education world:

in 2021, a hundred years after May applied to medical school, *U.S. News & World Report* ranked New York University number four and Columbia University number six in the category of best medical schools for research.[28] May would've happily accepted the offer to attend Flower Hospital's associated medical school, even though it practiced a sect of medicine that was quickly losing acceptance within the US. But with a mentor providing a slight course correction, May instead set her sights on two medical schools that are still considered some of the best in the US, and arguably the world.

Impressively, May was admitted to both schools. Columbia gave her a conditional acceptance; she would be allowed to join the medical class in the fall if she took a chemistry course over the summer. Medical schools still do this today. Unfortunately, this was a hurdle May couldn't surmount. She was already breaking her back to pay for college. Saving up for medical school just added to that burden. After graduating from college, she worked for a year in the pathology lab, and she needed every penny of that income to pay for medical school. She didn't have the luxury of taking time off over the summer to take the chemistry course. Thankfully, NYU didn't have the same prerequisite. She happily accepted NYU's offer and joined the entering class of 1922.

NYU maintained an unofficial quota, as did many medical schools, and May recalled that NYU usually accepted only two women. Her medical class was different. The school admitted five women. One female student was the daughter of a wealthy donor to the hospital. Another was the relative of one of the college's professors. A third was the highest-ranked undergraduate student at Hunter College. It took incredible circumstances like those for the school to willingly train more women than it had predetermined for its quota. The number of black students was also kept low. There were only four black students in the class, three of whom were men. May stood at the intersection of these two underrepresented groups: she was the only black woman in the group of five female students, and the only woman in the group of four black students.

Even more discouraging than the initial class demographics are the demographics of the graduating class. While all four of the white women graduated, the black men didn't fare as well. One of the black male students was discharged, and another died of tuberculosis. So on graduation day in 1926, only two black students remained to don their celebratory gowns: Dr. May Chinn and Dr. Aubre Maynard, who later became the chief surgeon of Harlem Hospital. They were the only two black students who made it to the end.

While Dr. Chinn remembers the clear racial discrimination that Dr. Maynard experienced in medical school due to his dark complexion, the most significant barrier she experienced was due to her financial constraints. Dr. Chinn worked throughout medical school in multiple labs, including Dr. Broadhurst's bacteriology lab and a clinical pathology lab at the New York State Department of Health.[29] She worked over summer break and during the school year. Of all the medical students I know at Penn and across the country, there are very few I know who are working while in medical school. And I can't think of anyone who works multiple jobs during the school year. If today's norms are any indicator, it was very unusual for a medical student to work during the school year. The demands of medical school were just too great.

The workload for a medical student today can give insight into what it was like to study medicine in the 1920s. Each day, students are responsible for attending hours of didactic lectures. This is just the first exposure to the material. They must digest the information so thoroughly that they can see the connections between multiple complex concepts. This level of understanding is necessary to apply the basic scientific ideas to dynamic clinical cases. To reach this level of comprehension, most students spend hours reviewing the material they have learned in the past few days. This is difficult for any student. But the task is much harder for a working student. May's intense schedule proved that.

Every day, she woke up around the time that the sun peeked into the sky. She was likely still sleepy when she got dressed and packed her bag for the day. Before eight in the morning, she scrambled to catch her bus. As the bus jumped from bumps in the road, medical facts hopped around in May's mind. This was her prime studying time. She would arrive at school by nine and file into the lecture hall with her classmates. There, she sat in on hours of lecture. Once that was finally done, she participated in labs, engaged in clinical visits, or studied new material. By six in the evening, she was out of the medical school, heading to the lab, say at the New York State Department of Health, for work. She remained in that windowless workspace until eleven at night. About five hours of research allowed for some solid experiments. Then, she used the moon in the sky and any streetlamps to navigate her way to the bus stop. She was trying to catch the Number 2 bus back home. If she felt up to it, she would fit in another study session. She must have gotten good at shutting out any rowdiness from her fellow passengers. By midnight, she'd arrive back home. Surely exhausted, May climbed into bed. She needed her energy to do all this again the next day.[30]

May had to be incredibly intelligent to get through medical school with this schedule. Nowadays, students often liken attending medical school to drinking out of a firehose. To me, it feels more like being a hamster running on a wheel, but at speeds comparable to those of marathon races in the Summer Olympics. We're constantly on the move. And when we're gasping for air, yearning to be done with the race, we take another turn and just keep going. Although it feels impossible for many when we're in the thick of it, we make it through. Still, to meet the intense demands of medical school while managing a twenty-five-hour-plus work week schedule? That sounds nothing short of miraculous.

One thing that likely helped her manage the hectic schedule was her background in clinical pathology. It afforded her skills that the typical medical student didn't have. For instance, she knew how to administer anesthesia to a patient, thanks to her experience giving anesthesia to animals. Her school's clinical pathology professor recognized her relative expertise in the field. He insisted that she serve as a student assistant for her classmates during their second year of medical school. Consider the cognitive dissonance May's classmates experienced when they realized they were going to learn this complex topic from not only a classmate but the sole black woman in their class. She was probably the last person they'd expect to have teach them anything.

Even as a black woman in medicine, I would be surprised at such a situation. My shock would come not from prejudiced beliefs about the capabilities of black women. Instead, I would be more surprised that a predominantly white medical institution would allow a black female medical student to have that kind of influence, even in the 2020s. In the 1920s, racist acts against African Americans were surging. There were numerous deadly Ku Klux Klan attacks in the US in the period after World War I.[31] Based on this social context, I would assume black women had fewer opportunities then than they do today. But almost one hundred years after Dr. Chinn completed her medical training, the percentage of black female medical educators is scant. In 2018, only 2 percent of all US medical faculty were black women, and only about 15 percent of those black women faculty were full professors.[32]

This discrepancy was made obvious to me during my first year of medical school. I was constantly exposed to new professors; physicians deemed experts on specific topics were selected to give talks. For example, different professors would lecture on childbirth and on cervical cancer. Despite this diversity of clinical topics, it wasn't until March 1, 2021, that a black physician delivered a lecture for my class. This was after more than six months of classes and having studied under more than 150 physician lecturers and lab preceptors. To me, this scenario signals who medical schools believe is competent enough to train the next generation of physicians, and who is not.

May's pathology professor likely had a small pool of people to choose from, since clinical pathology was an emerging field. Still, her appointment to this position may have challenged her classmates' preconceptions of the capabilities of black women. It showed that she was their intellectual equal, that she could hold her own in medicine. After four years of hard work and persistence, Dr. May Chinn graduated from New York University Medical College in 1926 as the school's first African American woman graduate.

After clearing one hurdle, Dr. Chinn immediately faced yet another. Following graduation, she experienced intense racial discrimination. Residency programs, a crucial step in postgraduate training, refused to admit her. Hospitals refused to hire her. Every black physician in Harlem faced this form of discrimination, but she was not deterred. To further her medical training, she worked for a group of male physicians who had a private practice at the Edgecombe Sanitarium on Edgecombe Avenue and 137th Street in New York City.

She was treated like the grunt worker of this practice. On call 24/7, Dr. Chinn was the one woken up in the middle of the night to care for the other doctors' patients. The other doctors treated Dr. Chinn like their personal servant, not their colleague. She endured long hours. Even worse, she experienced disrespectful attitudes from the doctors in the practice who didn't believe she should be a physician because she was a black woman. Some of the doctors didn't even acknowledge her presence. Dr. Chinn recalled, "One said that I didn't exist—you know; I just didn't exist."[33]

Despite all of Dr. Chinn's contributions to the private practice, the doctors rarely paid her for her clinical services. They went as far as making her pay rent to stay in the building that housed the office even though she was doing them a favor. The Department of Health required a physician to be a resident on the property. While physicians often cite residency as a particularly grueling stage of their training, Dr. Chinn's apprenticeship-like postgraduate training was made especially difficult by these harsh conditions.

Because Dr. Chinn was isolated from her community, her situation was even harder to cope with. She was the only black woman physician practicing in Harlem for many years. Though she faced similar challenges as the black male physicians, even some of them didn't support her. They looked down on her because she was a woman. When Dr. Chinn sought a job in public health, numerous black and white male physicians joined together to protest her hiring at the Department of Health. They said that they "didn't want to be tied to the apron strings of a woman."[34] Dr. Chinn stayed at the Edgecombe practice for twelve years because it was one of the only places where she could get substantial clinical work experience. She was finally pushed out from the clinic in the 1930s, when the other doctors increased rent to a point that she couldn't afford.

Dr. Chinn's next step was to open her own practice. To maintain the practice with her limited funds, innovation was essential. She treated patients who had been turned away by the regular hospitals. When a hospital turned away a black patient because of their race, the patient turned to Dr. Chinn. Japan's attack on the US Pacific Fleet at Pearl Harbor in Hawaii on December 7, 1941, prompted the formal entry of the United States into World War II the next day, and the conflict prompted many white doctors in New York City to turn away their Japanese patients. Dr. Chinn cared for those patients too.

The patients had a variety of ailments. Some needed surgery. In these situations, Dr. Chinn teamed up with Dr. Peter Marshall Murray, a trained surgeon from Howard University College of Medicine. Dr. Chinn described her medical practice as reminiscent of practices "a hundred years before."[35] When these two African American doctors entered a patient's home, they carefully surveyed the space. They needed to figure out how they were going to adapt the area for an antiseptic surgery. Depending on the size of the patient, the bed or an ironing board might be designated as the operating table. The presence of a coal stove was vital. The doctors would wrap up their dressings in newspapers and bake them in the oven. In less time than it took to bake a loaf of bread, the dressing was sterilized and safe to use. Then, Dr. Chinn or Dr. Murray would ask the family to show them to the washroom. The family's wash boiler, which usually washed clothes, could also disinfect their surgical instruments.

With their tools cleaned, the doctors' next step was finding light that was strong enough to give them a clear view during the surgery. The patients generally used kerosene lamps to light their homes. The fire in the center of a lamp's glass bowl lit the room only dimly. They needed something strong. Dr. Chinn and Dr. Murray decided to bring their office lamps with batteries to ensure enough lighting during surgery. With everything set up, Dr. Chinn would administer the anesthesia. Once a patient was stabilized, Dr. Murray would start the surgery.

Whenever a patient needed a blood transfusion, Dr. Chinn and Dr. Murray worked together against the clock. Dr. Chinn would conduct blood counts, blood typing, and urinalysis in a makeshift lab she had built in her home. Then they would prepare the blood donor, who oftentimes was a family member or a neighbor. Relying on direct transfusion, the doctors needed only a few small needle pokes for the blood to flow from the donor to the recipient. Dr. Chinn and Dr. Murray could complete the entire transfusion process within twelve hours.

Once the surgery was done, the two doctors took turns watching over the patient. They were both on call until the patient was able to get up. They didn't let their fatigue impair their clinical care. While it was risky to conduct a surgery without the help of a larger medical team, the doctors found support in the family. A patient's grandmother, or another family member, would serve as their nurse. With some help and a heap of innovation, these doctors were accomplishing the remarkable feat of providing care for patients who had been discarded by the medical system.

Over the course of her private practice, Dr. Chinn noticed a concerning trend among her older patients. In spite of great care from their family members, many appeared to be wasting away. Dr. Chinn suspected that they were afflicted by cancer. Many of these patients' cancers had progressed too far for Dr. Chinn to help them. All she could do was prescribe them medication to ease their pain. Wanting to, and believing she could, do more, Dr. Chinn dedicated herself to figuring out how to diagnose cancer earlier. This, in her view, was the key to better outcomes for her patients. In the 1940s, Sloan Kettering Institute, which is now known as the Memorial Sloan Kettering Cancer Center, was the only New York City hospital that studied cancer.[36] When Dr. Chinn had a patient who was well enough to walk on their own, she sent them to Memorial Hospital to be examined. Initially, they would be turned away. The hospital received a high volume of patients, and the black patients could not afford the hospital's fees. In response, Dr. Chinn started going to the clinic with her patients and requesting to watch the doctor examine them. The clinic did not always accept her requests, but on the few occasions when it did, Dr. Chinn was able to learn new techniques, which she added to examinations at her office.

One of the techniques that she learned was how to collect a biopsy—a tissue sample. She started obtaining biopsies from the patients she suspected might have cancer. Then, she sent the samples to the diagnostic section of Memorial Hospital. These samples would typically have been refused because she was a black physician, but she had a connection on the inside: some of the white male physicians at the hospital were her former classmates. They would accept her samples and analyze them for her. After Dr. Chinn had been doing this for about twelve years, black male physicians and white physicians finally started to recognize her expertise. They began referring their patients to her for biopsies. She would send the samples to Memorial with her name attached to them.

Thanks to her growing reputation, Dr. Chinn received a phone call from Dr. Elise L'Esperance, a white woman physician who founded the Kate Depew Strang Clinic for Cancer and Allied Diseases at the New York Infirmary, a cancer detection clinic in New York City. During this call, Dr. L'Esperance offered Dr. Chinn a position at her clinic. Dr. Chinn was shocked because black physicians were still excluded from working in clinics in the early 1940s. She tried to suspend her excitement until she met Dr. L'Esperance in person. Dr. Chinn suspected that Dr. L'Esperance assumed she was Chinese, based on Chinn's last name. Many had made that mistake before.

When Dr. Chinn showed up at the appointment, Dr. L'Esperance was shocked. She didn't expect a black woman to appear in her office. Dr. L'Esperance probably would not have offered Dr. Chinn the job if she had known that Dr. Chinn was African American. Thankfully, Dr. L'Esperance didn't rescind the offer once she found out. She might have had little choice because the number of white men practicing medicine at that time in the US had declined, as they were abroad serving in the war.

Dr. Chinn's racially ambiguous name had helped her sidestep some of the systematic discrimination she had experienced for much of her career, allowing her to be judged based on her credentials rather than negative stereotypes about her race. Dr. Chinn worked at Memorial Hospital from 1945 through 1976. After many years on the job, she was put in charge of three clinics, where nine white men and women physicians worked under her. It is unclear when she was appointed to these leadership positions, but social movements may have helped her climb the professional ladder. The civil rights movement and second-wave feminism occurred in the middle of her tenure at Memorial clinic. These

TWICE AS HARD • 37

movements altered the social landscape of the US and made it a bit easier for black Americans and women to ascend within their medical fields.

May had been born into an extremely disadvantaged family. For the daughter of an American slave to become a doctor in the early twentieth century is truly remarkable. Her parents had very little education, so they didn't know what she needed to do to be successful in the medical field. There were many moments when May's journey could have led her to have a very different life. As a young girl, she experienced the pressure to perform the supposed duties of a woman: get married and have children. The pressure indirectly led her to leave high school. Without a high school diploma or any higher education, May could have easily taken part in menial work that would have kept her in the same depressed socioeconomic situation that her parents were in.

Persistent encouragement from her mother eventually led May to resume her education. Once she got that second chance, she realized that she could achieve more than she had previously thought possible. Coming from a disadvantaged background, May needed champions like her mother and her college bacteriology professor to push her further to realize her potential. Once May earned her medical degree, other medical professionals who were racist and sexist tried to prevent her from succeeding in the profession. With limited resources and few opportunities to further her medical skills, Dr. Chinn had to be incredibly hardworking, creative, and resilient in order to succeed both as a physician and as the only black woman physician practicing in Harlem for many years. Her background is similar to that of many black women in her generation. With the numerous obstacles Chinn experienced, it's easy to see why there were so few black women physicians in the early twentieth century—and so remarkable to hear the story of a woman who broke through barriers throughout her life and left us with a legacy to admire and emulate.

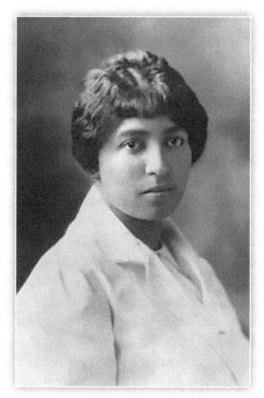

Dr. Dorothy Ferebee

CHAPTER 3

DOING GOOD IN THE COMMUNITY

Given the numerous structural barriers that choked the rate of new black women physicians at the turn of the twentieth century, the black women who were able to thrive in these barren conditions likely came from families whose support helped to make up for the societal oppression they faced. For many, this support was likely coupled with privilege—the familial privilege to help daughters dream of a future that entailed more than being a nanny or house cleaner for a white family, and the financial resources to help daughters make that dream a reality. Dorothy Celeste Boulding Ferebee was blessed to be raised in a family like this.

Born in Norfolk, Virginia, in 1898, two years after May Chinn, Dorothy was not afforded the dignity of knowing her birth date. She was born in a hospital that upheld racist practices. The doctors refused to issue a birth certificate for African American babies. This practice was commonplace throughout Norfolk. It's as if these medical institutions detested black life so much that they didn't want to recognize the beginning of new life. Dorothy's family tried to work against this dehumanizing practice by making note of when Dorothy entered the world. Their best guess for her birthday was October 10, 1898.

While Dorothy was brought up in a society that reinforced the idea that her life held little value due to her race and gender, she had a family who countered this false narrative. They were highly educated and accomplished black professionals. This was proof that Dorothy could find professional success too. Her family included lawyers and writers, and a judge. Their upward social mobility outpaced that of most African

Americans at the time. Still, their start in America was the same as May's family's and every other African American: through slavery.

Dorothy's parents were Benjamin Richard Boulding and Florence "Flossie" Cornelia Paige Boulding. The family wealth came from her mother's side. Dorothy's maternal grandfather, Richard Gault Leslie Paige, was born into slavery. He escaped when he was ten via the Underground Railroad. A local antislavery society in Boston aided in his escape. It helped him reunite with his aunt, who had escaped from slavery before him. As he grew into his freedom, Richard earned a living as a craftsman. Eventually, he became a Massachusetts state legislator. Dorothy's great-uncle, George L. Ruffin, carried on the family's tradition of black excellence when he became the first black person to graduate from Harvard Law School and went on to serve as first black judge in Massachusetts.[1]

Imagine being born into such a family legacy. She was a black girl in the early 1900s with so much stacked against her. She was also a black girl born into a family of extremely accomplished black people with strong connections in the community. I grew up as a black girl with successful parents, so I can understand the paradoxical situation she was in. She was engulfed in a society that tried to convince her that she wasn't smart or talented enough to make an impact. Yet, her family served as an inspirational cocoon that shielded her from these discouraging messages. This is the space where she developed her own dreams. Whenever someone told me that I wouldn't be successful in college or in a STEM career, I would just think of my parents. I believed that if they could succeed, I could too. It didn't matter that most of the African Americans on TV were depicted negatively, or that I knew only a handful of black people who were leaders in their fields. My parents' example as college-educated professionals was enough to encourage me to try. Maybe this was how Dorothy felt.

Dorothy developed an interest in medicine at a young age. Her ambitions, coupled with her mother falling ill, probably motivated her parents to move Dorothy to Boston to live with her great-aunt, Emma Ruffin. At this time, the intense levels of discrimination in southern states like Virginia likely stifled many black girls from achieving their dreams. While northeastern states like Massachusetts still had their problems, they offered many more opportunities for African Americans. By the time Dorothy moved to Boston, more than a hundred black women had trained at northeastern medical schools, while none had been allowed to study at predominantly white southern medical schools.[2] Dorothy completed most of her formal education in Boston. Privilege countered prejudice, giving Dorothy access to opportunities that most black children in her generation did not have. Without the opportunity to leave the South, another promising and ambitious black girl born at the same time in the same city likely wouldn't have become a physician.

Following a successful high school career, Dorothy started at Simmons College in the fall of 1916. Remaining focused on her medical aspirations, she bravely expressed this interest to a few of her professors. While it was common during this time for women to be discouraged from pursuing this path, the Simmons professors encouraged Dorothy to pursue her goal. They also connected her with various physicians at nearby Tufts University School of Medicine. Their support kept Dorothy motivated as she plowed through numerous challenging science courses. Toward the end of her time at Simmons, she applied to medical school. Dorothy started medical school at Tufts in the fall of 1920, only weeks after the Nineteenth Amendment to the US Constitution was ratified, granting women the right to vote, but almost five decades before black women were able to exercise this right throughout the US.[3]

Although Simmons and Tufts were only three miles apart, their cultures were vastly different. While the professors at Simmons were excited to see a black woman become a physician, many of the professors at Tufts had no interest in training women for careers in medicine. The attitude toward women in medicine at Tufts was evident in class makeup. In Dorothy's medical class of 143, only 5 students were women. Dorothy stood out as the only black woman in her class. These women accounted for only 3.5 percent of the class, but the percentage of female medical students was actually higher than normal. Dorothy believed that the school had an unofficial quota limiting enrollment to three women per class, similar to Dr. Chinn's suspicions about NYU.[4] The increased diversity of Dorothy's class was attributable to wealth and institutional connections: one female student was the daughter of a very wealthy banker, and another female student had family connections to the medical school. Dorothy's experience mirrored that of Dr. Chinn; it took extreme privilege and wealth to convince the white male faculty at Tufts to admit a few more women into the medical school. While Dorothy and her white female classmates had different ethnic and socioeconomic backgrounds, they found solace in one another as they navigated sexism at an overwhelmingly male medical school. This was not always the case for black women pursuing medicine.

When Dorothy started medical school, she held the logical expectation that her professors would give her medical training in exchange for the high tuition payments. Instead, the Tufts medical professors neglected Dorothy and the other female students. For the first three years, the instructors acted as if they didn't exist. Whether in a large auditorium with all their classmates or in smaller learning groups, the women were always passed over when opportunities for individual learning arose. When a woman raised her hand in class, lecturers pretended they couldn't see her. Anytime there was an opportunity for a student to give a presentation, male students were the only ones selected.

This gender-based exclusion persisted in the clinics. When students began to practice delivering diagnoses at the bedside, a necessary skill to be a competent physician, none of the five women were permitted to give the diagnosis. They were even relegated to clinical experiences that aligned more with a nursing curriculum, such as the bandage clinic or the foot-soaking clinic. In comparison, the male students had extensive exposure to the clinics most applicable to physicians, such as the surgery and medical clinics. Despite all of these obstacles, the women refused to allow bigotry to impede their dreams. In a 1979 interview, Dorothy reflected on how they persisted in those times: "The five of us decided that we would stick together, and we would study together, and we would outrun some of these difficulties surrounding us."[5] The mutual support and encouragement were necessary when they wanted to cry tears of sorrow or scream out in frustration over their situation.

But once these women reached their third year of medical school, they deemed the disadvantages in medical training too great to endure in silence. That year, their medical class had the opportunity to receive clinical training at Massachusetts General Hospital, a world-class teaching hospital associated with Harvard Medical School. Every Friday afternoon, from one to five, the students would crowd into the hospital's amphitheater and watch as a well-regarded physician presented complex clinical cases. After providing key details about a case, the physician would choose a few lucky medical students to work through the case systematically. What is your differential diagnosis? How would you go about elucidating the true cause of the patient's chief complaint? What is the proper treatment plan for this patient? Practice working up a clinical case in this fashion is vital for any budding physician.

But in this room filled with promising physicians in training, the five women were treated differently. Dorothy described how her professor made her feel: "We could've really been dust on the wall or a spot on the floor as far as he was concerned because he never even looked at us."[6] Imagine how difficult it must have been for these women to be treated as if they were worthless, by an accomplished physician and possible role model. It would've been easy for them to internalize this man's prejudice and believe that they didn't belong in the space, wondering if maybe the admissions committee made a mistake when it had admitted them. But Dorothy and her friends knew the truth. They had earned their spots in medical school just as fully as their male classmates had.

In the fall of their third year, the women marched into the office of the dean of students for Tufts Medical School. While reporting the Harvard-affiliated physician put students in a very vulnerable position, they mustered up enough courage to speak truth to power. The women were upfront with the dean about the professor's discriminatory treatment, and they emphatically explained how the professor's behavior was impacting their medical educations. The dean listened attentively. He appeared sympathetic to their plight. After learning more details about the situation, he promised to do something to fix the problem. The women waited eagerly to see how the dynamic in the hospital would change. As weeks passed by, it became clear that either the dean had done nothing to remedy the situation or his actions were not persuasive enough to convince the Mass General physician to actually acknowledge the women in his class.

The women may have felt discouraged when they realized that the dean of students would not protect them from a professor's discriminatory behavior, but they knew they had power within themselves. They resolved to work together to fill the gaps in their clinical knowledge and skills. They agreed to meet every Friday and Saturday to discuss cases from five foreign medical journals that they deemed important: from Vienna, Paris, Berlin, England, and Scotland. They would explain the different clinical cases and the medical teams' therapeutic approaches. By sampling such a large array of cases, the women were more than prepared for the sessions at Mass General Hospital, as well as those in their clinics.

Solidarity was vital in keeping the study group together. One of the students was Polly, a Jewish woman. She had difficulty attending the Friday sessions because she was expected to observe her faith's Sabbath from sundown on Friday to sundown on Saturday. During that period, she was expected to rest—not engage in work, like studying. After reflecting on how she practiced her faith, she decided that she wanted to join the study group, but she needed permission from her rabbi. She explained her plight to her friends. The other four women offered to accompany Polly to a discussion with the rabbi. The five women met with the rabbi and described the unique challenges they were up against in medical school, and how their study group had been formed to ensure that all five of them completed their medical educations. The rabbi saw the importance of their efforts, so he allowed Polly to participate in the weekend study sessions.

Mary, a daughter of Italian immigrants, and Marguerite Kelly, a member of a staunch Irish Catholic family, also faced cultural obstacles in their communities. Just as they had banded together to speak with Polly's rabbi, the women joined forces to convince Mary's and Marguerite Kelly's families of the importance of the work they were doing. Following these conversations, both women were allowed to participate in the study group. Luckily, Dorothy didn't have any issues gaining family support to participate in the group. Dorothy's great-aunt Emma, along with the rest of Dorothy's family, were extremely enthusiastic about Dorothy's pursuit of a medical degree. Her great-aunt Emma encouraged Dorothy and her friends to study any day they needed. She even offered her home as a study spot.

On a brisk winter afternoon in early February, the students finally had a chance to correct their professor's false perceptions of them. As on many Friday afternoons before, an orderly rolled a patient into the auditorium. The professor instructed the orderly to undrape the patient and carefully place him on the clinic table. Then, without looking at any of the women, he called all five of them by their last names and announced that he wanted them to take charge of the case.

Hearing the sound of her name made Dorothy feel breathless. She was ecstatic to finally be acknowledged by her professor. The professor may have seen this as an opportunity to embarrass the female medical students, but they weren't afraid. They had studied for countless hours. They were ready to put their hard work to the test. The professor instructed an intern to read a clinical vignette about the patient to the medical students. Dorothy listened to the description of the patient's primary illness and information on how long he had been afflicted by it, and a host of other details. As the intern laid out the case, a light went off in Dorothy's head. The case bore a strong resemblance to a case from the Vienna journal article that the five women had reviewed a couple of weeks earlier. The other four women were in sync with Dorothy about the connection between the cases. It was a complicated case, but the women understood it well. Still, they remained calm and didn't reveal the added confidence that now surged through them.

Once the history had been read, the professor asked the women to speak. With so much time spent reviewing cases, the women knew one another's strengths. While the first woman reviewed the patient's chief complaint and obtained a family medical history, the next woman followed up with a physical exam. Dorothy remembered noting that none of the men in the room were paying attention to their extremely thorough work, but she remained focused. The next woman presented her differential diagnosis. To narrow down the list of potential diagnoses, she requested various labs.

After the group of women had reviewed the lab results, physical exam outcome, and history, Dorothy was elected to give the final diagnosis. Dorothy stood tall, as the only black woman in a room full of white men who refused to treat her as an equal. Then she gave a case summary that was impossible to ignore. She went through each diagnosis that was high on her team's differential, laid out the clinical findings that supported a given diagnosis, and pointed out any evidence that would persuade her against a particular diagnosis. After providing thorough arguments against various diagnoses, Dorothy delivered her final diagnosis. The professor—who was not expecting the women to figure out the correct diagnosis—stood with his mouth opened, in shock. He became angered that his attempt to humiliate the five women with a difficult case was unsuccessful. His blood began to boil and he went red behind the ears. He decided to target his rage at Dorothy. After avoiding eye contact throughout the entire presentation, he chose this moment to finally look Dorothy in the eye. But instead of showing respect or pride at her adept handling of the case, he had fire in his eyes. In front of the entire class, he thundered: "So you think you're pretty good, don't you?"[7]

She knew that he expected her to acquiesce. He wanted her to say something indicating that she did not believe that she was smart or impressive. Dorothy was not a person who would typically challenge a professor, but she had reached her breaking point. This man had ignored her and her friends for months, and now attempted to challenge their intelligence with a case he deemed impossible for them to solve. So instead of submitting to his bigotry, Dorothy confidently rebutted: "Sir, I don't think I'm pretty good. I think I'm *very* good."[8] To this response, the whole amphitheater went wild in support of her. The men clapped vigorously. Some stamped their feet. They had been converted from seriously doubting the five women's capabilities to being completely impressed with their intellects and dedication to medicine. The doctor was outraged by the positive response to the women. He abruptly turned away from the crowd and charged out the door.

Dorothy marked the day as the moment the five women were finally considered part of the class of 1924. Their male classmates finally respected them. The men began consulting the women on various clinical cases. The men recognized that not only were these women their equals, but they had insights that the men could learn from. After three years of trekking through the trenches of medical school as students who were alienated from much of their class, the five women were finally accepted as members of the community. At the end of their medical schooling, all five women graduated with honors and were ranked among the top 9 of 143 in the class.

After graduating from medical school, Dr. Dorothy Boulding was asked by various organizations to speak at events throughout the country. Sometimes her friends from medical school would attend the events. In an interview, she reflected on the experience: "[When] they ask me to speak to public groups, I'll always say that the five women were among the first nine. And then one of them will jump up. Polly will jump up and say, 'Well I want to correct something that Dorothy Boulding had said. She isn't telling the truth. . . . Yes, the five women were in the top nine, but she never tells anybody that she was number one.' So, in a class of 143 people, I was first. But I never bragged about it. I let my colleagues tell the story."[9]

When Tufts medical students were still in their final year of medical school, they began preparing for the next steps, sending their residency applications to various programs around the country. Unfortunately, the bigotry that the women faced at Tufts played out on a national scale. Dr. Dorothy Boulding faced the brunt of it. The entire medical class submitted residency applications around the same time, but the residency programs delivered responses in phases. Early into the students' final year, all the men had been accepted into residency programs. The women likely felt anxious while the men received their placements because the women still hadn't even been acknowledged by the programs they applied to.

Finally, in May, months after the men were sure of their next steps, responses for the women began to filter in. Sadly, the letters brought disappointment. They made excuses: "I'm sorry, the application list has been filled," or "I'm sorry, we are not taking women this year."[10] One residency program even told Dr. Boulding that her academic record was not strong enough for its program. If a woman ranked number one in her medical class at a well-regarded medical school isn't good enough, what is? Unsurprisingly, the men ranked below her were considered strong enough applicants to qualify for residency programs.

Residency programs likely sent similar letters to other female applicants across the country. These applicants had to find ways to attain postgraduate clinical training, or they wouldn't be able to become licensed physicians. The white women in Dr. Boulding's class used their family connections and wealth to gain admission to residency programs. Dr. Boulding's family didn't have that kind of social capital, but they refused to let her career aspirations vanish. Her brother found a way to help.

Dorothy's oldest brother, Ruffin Paige Boulding, had gained admission to Howard University School of Law. Located in Washington, DC, Howard is a historically black university committed to training black people from the university level to professional school. Unfortunately, the cost of attendance was more than Ruffin could afford. But he was determined, like his sister. He delayed his own education and took a job in Boston to raise enough money for his tuition. After many years, he had saved enough money to finally go to school. Around this time, he learned of Dorothy's struggles to find a residency placement. Ruffin was familiar with the opportunities in DC. He gave Dorothy insight on how to navigate the system. She would need to travel to DC and take an exam, which would make her eligible for a spot at a government hospital. Ruffin knew that Dorothy had her own financial constraints due to the costs of medical school and living in Boston. He didn't want lack of money to impede her success, so he used money from his savings to buy her a train ticket. He told her that if she had challenges affording housing in Washington, he would take the next year off to ensure that she could complete her residency training.

She took her older brother's advice and traveled to Washington to complete the exam. Given its more objective nature, the written exam was easy for Dr. Boulding to pass. Things grew more complicated during the oral exam, which was conducted by a panel of white men with their own agenda. They wanted their sons to receive the medical internship placement, and Dr. Boulding was a threat to their nepotistic practices. They also told Dr. Dorothy Boulding that they didn't see why any woman should be selected for the internship position, regardless of her credentials. This constant rejection must have been extremely frustrating for Dr. Boulding. It didn't matter how hard she worked. If the gatekeepers of medicine didn't want her in the field, she couldn't join.

Despite this committee's persistent corruption, one of the physicians took pity on Dr. Boulding because of her situation. He was familiar with Howard University and its teaching hospital, Freedmen's Hospital. He encouraged Dr. Boulding to investigate opportunities at the predominantly black hospital, rather than seek a place at a predominantly white government hospital. She was referred to Dr. William A. Warfield Jr., the superintendent of the hospital. Dr. Warfield was impressed by Dr. Boulding's credentials and interview, so he offered her a residency position at Freedmen's Hospital. Dr. Dorothy Boulding began her residency training in the summer of 1924.

Dr. Boulding was so grateful for the opportunity to further her clinical education that she prioritized it over many things in her personal life. Her home was the hospital. Her black male co-residents enjoyed their weekends at baseball games or dances, but Dr. Boulding didn't indulge in such luxuries. She oftentimes found herself in the hospital on Saturdays and Sundays, accompanied only by one or two other interns of the eleven in her class. By the time she completed her internship year, she had experience in every ward, even though she hadn't been assigned to them all.

One aspect of her clinical training involved serving with the crews of Freedmen's ambulances in the late 1920s. Her ambulance was frequently called to care for people who had been wounded in street fights or domestic disturbances in southeast Washington. Due to redlining, many of the African Americans from low-income backgrounds were segregated to this area. During this time, Dr. Boulding saw more than just broken bones. She saw the challenges that the community faced, which improved her understanding of the people's social needs.

One issue that really struck her was the lack of opportunities for children. Many of the schools were rundown. The city government deprived the predominantly black school district of funds that it freely distributed to the nearby white school districts. As a result, black school-age children's academic progress was blunted, compared to that of their peers. Younger children were in an even more precarious position. They were left at home when their mothers went to work (sometimes as early as five in the morning). Mothers tried to enlist caretakers to watch over their children, but the mothers' finances were strained. Caretakers were usually a grandmother or older sibling.

Dr. Boulding recalled a similar dynamic in the neighborhood where she lived. One woman would take care of multiple children on her block while their mothers and fathers went to work. Even with all hands on deck, the families struggled to make ends meet. As Dr. Boulding's nights on the ambulance wore on, she continued to see the challenges in the community. She became convinced that something needed to be done to help the people. She just wasn't sure what.

One day she was working in her office at a Freedmen's clinic when her phone rang. Expecting a call from a patient or colleague, Dr. Boulding was surprised to hear a police officer on the other end. This event was so memorable, she recalled details from it in an interview fifty years later: "This is the police department. This is Precinct Five over on Fifth Street and Southeast. We have a little boy here that we've arrested, and he says that you know him."

Startled, Dr. Boulding tried to elicit more information from the police officer. Instead of giving her more details, the officer insisted that she come over to the department. Dr. Boulding hurriedly closed out what she was working on and headed out the door. She jumped into her sleek two-seater, which her uncle had gifted her for graduating from medical school, and drove with her heart in her stomach until she finally arrived at the precinct. Once she reached the front desk, she implored: "What is this? What is this?"

Behind the desk, there was a little black boy with a runny nose and tears streaming down his face. He cried out to her: "Dr. Boulding, they're going to put me in jail!"

When she questioned the white policeman, who was hovering above the child, the policeman retorted, "Well he's been stealing!"

The little boy wailed in defense, "I wasn't stealing. I was getting some milk for my baby brother. He was crying and had no food. And momma had gone to work."

Dr. Boulding then asked the boy, "Does momma usually go to work and leave the baby?"[11]

The boy explained that his mother had to leave at six in the morning to go to work, leaving him to care for his two-year-old brother. At some point, the child began to cry. The little boy must have felt overwhelmed with the responsibility of taking care of a baby when he was still a child himself. He thought food might ease his little brother's distress. But when he went to the icebox for some food, he saw there was none. No milk. Not even any ice. Suddenly, the little boy felt hungry too. This hopeless situation filled him with sorrow, so he began to weep alongside the searing cries of his baby brother. He looked out his front door and saw that the milkman had just delivered a quart of milk to the family across the street. As soon as the milkman turned the corner, the little boy ran across the street and took the quart of milk. Before he could reach his house, a police officer appeared and dragged him to the police station.

When Dr. Boulding heard the full story, she was infuriated by how the child had been treated. She pleaded his case to the officers. One of the officers was very hostile. He didn't care what situation had led the child to take the milk. Thankfully, another officer was more sympathetic, so Dr. Boulding worked with him. They agreed that she could take the child and the milk to feed both children. In exchange, she paid for the milk, which at the time was about seventeen cents per quart. When they arrived at the boy's home, they found the baby extremely distraught. He was still crying and had torn up his bed. Since the officer had brought the boy to the precinct without allowing him to go home first, the two-year-old had been left alone for hours. This traumatic experience may have had a long-term psychological impact on the child.

Dr. Boulding fed both children and tried to soothe them. The disturbing situation left her uneasy. She waited with the kids until their mother returned home that evening. The mother had no idea what had happened to her children that day. She had brought leftover food from her job to stock the icebox. Dr. Boulding turned the children over to their mother and walked home. As she passed one block after another, she tried to process what had happened that day.

She recognized the societal dynamics that forced mothers to leave their children when they went to work. She also saw that children were at risk without a structured day care system. They could be neglected, or even face jail time for doing what they could to survive. Reflecting on the situation compounded the young doctor's initial yearning to help the community. She set her heart on helping to support the mothers and children struggling within this system. She knew there were day care centers in the area, but they refused to care for black children. So Dr. Boulding began work to create a day care that would care for black children in the area. Through this upsetting experience, the Southeast Settlement House was born.

Dr. Boulding applied for and received approximately nine thousand dollars from the local United Way foundation and other philanthropic organizations. She used the money to rent a six-room house, which became the day care center, and to hire people to help with the endeavor. Following extensive planning and organization, Dr. Boulding opened the Southeast Settlement House. At the time, it was the only day care serving black children in that part of DC. It slowly expanded to support more children. After-school programs were developed to get older children off the streets. By the late 1970s, the Southeast House served children, teenagers, and senior citizens. In addition to its initial services, it provided youth counseling, youth employment training, juvenile restitution, tutoring services, geriatric day care, and more. It served people living between South Capitol Street and the Anacostia River. Dr. Boulding noted the center was serving more than twelve thousand people in 1979. Its proposed budget for 1980 was $2.1 million.[12] Dr. Boulding built this incredible institution while she was completing her residency training. It continued to have a positive impact in the community through the early 1990s, more than sixty years after its founding.

Dr. Boulding's hard work in and out of the hospital caught the eye of Freedmen's Hospital superintendent, Dr. Warfield. When Dr. Boulding completed her residency, Dr. Warfield offered her a job as a professor in obstetrics at Howard University College of Medicine, with the option to also maintain her own private medical practice. In 1929, she was hired as a physician to women at the Howard University Health Service.

During her time at the health service, she met a handsome man named Dr. Claude Ferebee, who taught at Howard's College of Dentistry.

Claude was initially impressed by Dorothy's work at the university and the Southeast House. The two first became friends, thanks to their mutual respect for each other's work. Later, a strong attraction caused their friendship to blossom into something more romantic. They eventually married in 1930, prompting Dr. Boulding to change her name to Dr. Dorothy Boulding Ferebee.

They opened a joint medical and dental private practice a year after they tied the knot. At the same time, they started a family. By the end of 1931, Dorothy was pregnant with twins. Suddenly Dr. Ferebee had to balance the responsibilities of her job and the Southeast House plus the obligations that came with having a husband and two kids. While she loved all of these pursuits, her children held a special place in her heart, and she prioritized quality time with them over her work. She would typically read bedtime stories to her children when they were young. If story time conflicted with patients wanting to be seen, she would have her patients wait a bit. Being a mother had its challenges, but Dr. Ferebee found it extremely rewarding.

When the Great Depression hit in the 1930s, Dr. Ferebee felt a new drive to serve her community. The economic downturn devastated many communities in America, particularly the most vulnerable. She knew that many African Americans throughout the country were hit hard, and she wanted to do something to help them. Alpha Kappa Alpha Sorority became her avenue for having an impact. Founded in 1908, it was the first sorority for black college-educated women. Previously, there were white sororities throughout colleges in the US, but they did not allow black women to join. Alpha Kappa Alpha became an essential community for innumerable black women in the US and abroad. It boasts countless notable members, including Rosa Parks, Coretta Scott King, Toni Morrison, Mae Jemison, and Vice President Kamala Harris. Dorothy became a member of Alpha Kappa Alpha in the mid-1920s, while she was completing her medical degree. I also had the privilege of joining this wonderful organization, in 2016, following in my mother's footsteps. I have found sisters through the organization who have given me great joy and have inspired me to be my best self. Since starting medical school, I've been pleasantly surprised by the fact that many of my black female mentors in medicine are also members of my sorority.

Service has always been a central tenet of Alpha Kappa Alpha. We implement community outreach projects on the local, national, and international levels. Most of our projects aim to uplift the black community. Dr. Ferebee led one of these projects: Alpha Kappa Alpha's Mississippi Health Project. She served as the program's director from 1935 to 1941. The program focused on Bolivar County, a predominantly African American community that was struggling during the Great Depression. Like numerous other African American communities in the Jim Crow South, the people of Bolivar County suffered from dismal health facilities. A significant portion of Bolivar County's black men suffered from syphilis. This is one reason why the US Public Health Service selected Bolivar County, in addition to five other rural counties in the South, for the infamous Tuskegee experiment from 1932 to 1972.[13] Some of the same black men who were forced to live with untreated syphilis for decades may have also been Dr. Ferebee's patients. Residents of Bolivar County also frequently suffered from dysentery, and many died of tuberculosis.

Starting in the summer of 1935, Dr. Ferebee went to Mississippi with a team of African American women doctors, nurses, and teachers, many of whom were likely members of the sorority. From the start of their journey, these black women faced discrimination. They were volunteers from around the country who met in DC with the intention of taking a train down to Mississippi together. African Americans were allowed to ride only at the back of the train, in the Jim Crow car. The area was extremely hot and dirty. When Dr. Ferebee told the salesperson at the railway station that she wanted to buy seventeen tickets for herself and the other volunteers, he refused her request. There were only twenty-four seats open to black passengers, and the salesperson didn't want one group to take up so many of the seats. As a result, members of Dr. Ferebee's team were forced to drive their cars more than fifteen hours from DC to Bolivar County.

Once the women arrived in Mississippi, they faced hostility from the white plantation owners. These men didn't like the idea of black women coming to their area to provide healthcare. They initially denied the women's requests to access their workers. But eventually one plantation owner cosigned the sorority's efforts. With his encouragement, the other white men grudgingly allowed the black women to open a clinic. Dr. Ferebee and her team set up five clinics around the county. They had their medical instruments, medications, and a large supply of diphtheria and smallpox vaccines ready to care for the community.[14] On the day they opened, the clinics were eerily empty. They had notified the African Americans living in the community, but no one came. After further investigation, the women found out that many people wanted to come, but the plantation owners would not let the African Americans take a break from picking cotton in order to tend to their health. Unwilling to give up, the women declared, "Well, if they can't come to us, we'll go to them."[15] This is how the first mobile health clinic in the country was born.

These black women went to each plantation, carrying their medical supplies in their cars. Like Dr. Crumpler, who went to Richmond, Virginia, to provide medical care for recently freed African Americans, these black women were committed to serving a people whose health was generally ignored by American society. Alpha Kappa Alpha's Mississippi Health Project provided immunizations against diphtheria and smallpox to more than 14,000 children. It also treated thousands of adults for diseases that plagued the Bolivar community, such as malaria and syphilis. The black sharecroppers in the county also suffered from extreme malnutrition, so the team spent extensive time teaching families how to use their limited food supplies to correct malnutrition.[16] Dr. Ferebee's contribution to the health project garnered her support within the sorority, and in 1940, she became the Supreme Basileus (a.k.a. the national president) of Alpha Kappa Alpha Sorority, a role she held until 1951. She was the organization's first and only Supreme Basileus to date who was a physician.

Unfortunately, as Dr. Dorothy Ferebee saw increasing success in her career, her husband encountered challenges in his. This put a strain on their marriage. Around 1935, Dr. Claude Ferebee lost his faculty position at Howard, while she maintained her strong standing there. Dr. Dorothy Ferebee recounted the difficulties this caused with her husband. "He was becoming more and more resentful of everything that I was doing as a woman, because what I attempted seemed to turn to gold, and his effort was turning to mud. . . . That didn't set too well with him. And for that reason, he became very, shall I say, not disgruntled, but unhappy and uncooperative, and insisted that I give up my work. Of course, I wasn't going to do that."[17]

Dr. Dorothy Ferebee faced countless obstacles set by men who sought to hinder her success. She was finally reaching the peak of her career, but her husband wanted her to give it all up just to stroke his ego. To make matters worse, Claude betrayed their marital union by taking on multiple mistresses. Dorothy was left to cope with her husband's actions while caring for young twins and working a demanding job. Dorothy knew that if she refused her husband's demand to give up her job, more marital distress would ensue. Still, she held on to the unwavering determination that had helped her reach such high levels of success in the face of staunch sexism and racism. She told her husband no. She would not be hindered professionally, not even by her husband. Claude was too stuck on wanting a woman who would submit to his whims, so he allowed his resentment toward Dorothy's success to fester. He moved to New York, leaving his wife and kids behind.

Although this must have been painful for Dorothy, she found respite in her children and her professional life. The widespread impact that she had in the community caught the eye of Dr. Mordecai Wyatt Johnson, the first African American president of Howard University. He took her on as a mentee and encouraged her to strive for more. With his support and encouragement, Dr. Ferebee was named medical director of Howard University Health Services in 1949. This was noteworthy because it was almost unheard of for a woman to hold a high-level leadership position over men. Even at Howard University, a school that worked against racism, Dr. Ferebee saw sexism persist.[18] Many of the male physicians and directors at Howard resented Dr. Ferebee for her appointment as medical director. It is likely that she experienced further ostracization when the health division of the State Department selected her as a US representative for various global initiatives. It sponsored her for numerous medical service trips in Africa, Asia, and Europe.

While engaged in these global initiatives, Dr. Ferebee continued to expand her impact on the national stage. She became a visiting professor in preventive medicine at her alma mater, Tufts University School of Medicine. From 1949 to 1953, she was the president of the National Council of Negro Women. In 1950, she was appointed to the executive committee for the White House Conference on Children and Youth. She was also on the board of directors for various organizations, such as the Young Women's Christian Association and the Girl Scouts of the USA.

Amid all this success, tragedy struck. One of Dr. Ferebee's twins, Dorothy Ferebee Jr., fell ill. She had an infection that quickly overtook her body. She died suddenly in 1950, when she was only eighteen years old. The elder Dorothy struggled with the loss of her only daughter; her heart was broken. Leading up to this point, Dr. Dorothy Ferebee had been traveling between Washington, DC, and New York to maintain a relationship with her husband, despite their separation. Sadly, the loss of their daughter was the final crack in their marriage. Claude asked for a divorce, and Dorothy acceded to his request. Although she never fully recovered from the loss of her daughter, she buried herself in her work to cope.

In the 1960s, Dr. Ferebee was appointed to President Kennedy's American Food for Peace Council. She also became a medical consultant to the Peace Corps and to the State Department. She even spoke before the World Health Assembly in Geneva, Switzerland. Throughout all of this, she continued to build Howard's Health Services as its medical director, a position she held until 1968. That year, she was appointed medical associate to the dean of the College of Medicine at Howard University. In 1972, she retired from her private practice and her post at Howard.

Like Drs. Crumpler and Chinn, Dr. Dorothy Ferebee entered the medical field at a time when multiple structural barriers had been put in place to limit the number of black women in the profession. She prevailed in these hostile conditions by relying on her determination and grit, as well as the support of her family and a small group of peers and advisors who saw past her race and gender. In the 1920s, all women experienced intense sexism, so they developed tight-knit groups, irrespective of racial differences. Experiences from current medical students suggest that the level of solidarity that Dr. Ferebee enjoyed may not have persisted to the present, which is a loss to all of us.

Once Dr. Ferebee secured her place within medicine, she turned her focus to serving communities in need. Her involvement in Alpha Kappa Alpha Sorority helped her find other black women in medicine, many of them sharing her commitment to giving back. She worked with the sorority and multiple other service organizations to care for the underserved. Through her efforts, she positively impacted hundreds of thousands of lives and even had a global reach.

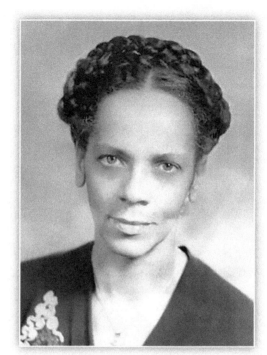

Dr. Lena Edwards

CHAPTER 4

FROM HER FAMILY FORWARD

Legacy is an enduring tenet of the culture of medicine. I remember, during one of my accepted students days at Harvard Medical School, an admissions officer tried to dispel feelings of imposter syndrome among the recent admits, saying, "It doesn't matter if your great-grandfather went to Harvard Medical School or if you're the first person in your family to attend medical school, each of you earned your place here at HMS." I was not feeling much imposter syndrome at the time, but I remember being struck by this concept. My great-grandfather was a sharecropper in Mississippi; it hadn't fully occurred to me that other medical students might have great-grandparents who had attended this very school ahead of them. I will be the first doctor in my family.

I had been so excited to participate in this admitted students' weekend. Gaining admission to Harvard Medical School still felt surreal. I needed to be on the medical campus to feel like I had truly been accepted. But in late February 2020, medical schools canceled their in-person admitted students days one by one, as the COVID-19 pandemic began to ravage the country, and the world. When I received notice that Harvard's in-person admitted students day was cancelled, I was devastated. I was struggling to choose between Harvard, Penn, and Columbia, and I was counting on the in-person events to help me discern which school felt right for me. Instead, I would have to rely on information gained during virtual events to make my final decision. As I sat in my living room watching Harvard's virtual admitted students' weekend on Zoom, the magic that surrounded this elite institution dissipated. It was just another school. Just another Zoom call.

But still, I had made it. Both my great-grandma and my grandma wanted to become physicians, but neither could because they didn't have the support to navigate the process or the money to finance it. I had much more support. But finances did influence my final decision. Harvard offered me limited financial aid, while Penn and Columbia offered me generous scholarships. Choosing Harvard meant signing on to more than $300,000 in debt. And while many students accepted this deal to become affiliated with Harvard's brand, it was a crushing burden that I could not bear. I had dreamed of attending HMS for six years, but I realized that I'd be much happier at Penn, where I'd gain an amazing education while securing a future with financial freedom.

As I made my decision, I assumed that the family legacies of students attending Harvard would be much different from those of students attending Penn. I figured there were only a few families with the generational wealth to support training multiple generations of doctors at elite institutions, and that those families would be clustered at Harvard Med. But when I matriculated at the Perelman School of Medicine at the University of Pennsylvania, I saw the same phenomenon. At a top-ten medical school like mine, it is common for more than half of the members of the class to have at least one parent who is a doctor. On a national level, one in five medical students has at least one parent who is a doctor.[1] Those who don't have a doctor as a parent are likely to have parents in some other high-paying profession. Nationally, approximately half of all entering medical students come from families in the richest twentieth percentile of the population. This demographic has never dipped below 48 percent of the entering medical school population since 1987, but the number of entering students from the lowest quintile of household income has never been above 5.5 percent.[2] This disproportionality is not the fault of the students with more privileged backgrounds. The medical school admission process and the requirements for successful completion of medical school favor applicants from wealthier backgrounds and with personal connections to physicians.[3] For African American applicants, whose families have faced generational oppression leading to disproportionately lower average education levels and household incomes, the journey to medical school is more difficult due to the systemic flaws in the process required to be admitted and then eventually to complete medical school.

When the Harvard admin gave us a fifteen-minute break between Zoom sessions, I sat back in my favorite armchair and took stock of my African American friend group. While many of them had parents who had bachelor's degrees and professional degrees, none had parents who were doctors. I guess it makes sense. Less than 2 percent of the physician population is black, so African American premedical students with parents in medicine would be few and far between. But what if an African American applicant did come from a long family lineage of doctors? Would her family's affluence override the challenges that would come her way due to race- and gender-based bigotry? If I had had a great-grandmother who was a doctor, what would she have had to go through to gift me with such an honorable family legacy? Dr. Lena Edwards shows me what it may have been like for my imaginary great-grandma.

Lena Edwards was born on September 17, 1900. Like Dorothy Boulding, Lena was raised in an affluent family. While neither of their parents were medical doctors, their family's money helped Lena and Dorothy jump through many of the hoops that aspiring physicians are still leaping through today. Lena's father, Thomas W. Edwards, earned his bachelor's degree from Howard University in 1887. Thomas was well ahead of his time. More than fifty years later, in 1940, less than 5 percent of all Americans twenty-five years or older had earned a bachelor's degree.[4] At the time Thomas earned his degree, the proportion of Americans with a bachelor's degree was likely substantially lower. Although Thomas was among the most educated men in the US, the best job he was able to obtain was at his local post office.

Thomas may have resentfully accepted being overqualified and underpaid when he was caring just for himself and his wife. By the time Lena was born, the family had expanded to five, with three young children, and Thomas didn't want his babies to grow up uncertain of when they would have their next meal. He strategized on how to game a system that was stacked against him. Eventually, he realized his alma mater,

Howard, was the answer. An institution dedicated to giving African Americans opportunities that they were so frequently denied, Howard was crucial to providing many members of the community access to professional degrees, which facilitated their social mobility. Twenty years after Thomas graduated from college, he went back to Howard to complete a dental degree.

At this point, he couldn't fall short on his responsibilities to his growing family. He endured countless exhausting days to strike this balance. He'd wake up early and trek to campus just in time for his first class. After many hours of lectures and labs, where he worked with dental drills and fillings, his eyes may have felt heavy. But once his classes were done, he must have spent some time studying his class material before heading to work. The moon shone high above the post office, a reminder that he should be in bed right now. After working a long shift, he would head home and sleep for a few hours, hoping to wake reenergized before he did it all over again. Finally, in 1907, when he was probably in his early forties, Thomas Edwards earned his dental degree from Howard University. A few years later, he joined the faculty at Howard University to pass on the gift of education to other African Americans.

Lena was only a little girl, but she saw how hard her dad was working to support the family and make a difference in their community. She admired his determination to give to others even at times when he was struggling himself. This is how she wanted to be when she grew up. When she spoke to him about her desire to follow in his footsteps and become a dentist, he expressed his concerns that her energetic personality might not be suited for dentistry. She took heed of his concerns and changed course slightly, fixing her eyes on medicine. Inheriting his determined spirit, Lena decided at eleven years old that she would become a physician, and that's exactly what she became. Even when she was young, she was aware that this aspiration went against the norm. In a 1977 interview, she reflected on this: "It was rather unusual for a woman, of all a black woman, to talk about being a doctor. . . . But I made up my mind I was going to be that, and that's what I wanted to be."[5] If her father wouldn't let the challenges associated with being an older black man with a wife and three kids prevent him from becoming a dentist, she wouldn't let the obstacles placed in front of her as a black woman prevent her from becoming a physician.

In addition to encouraging persistence, Lena's father helped her cultivate a sense of commitment to the black community, which was deepened by her proximity to the influential Carter G. Woodson, PhD. At the time Woodson was establishing an organization dedicated to African American history, founding the *Journal of Negro History*, and establishing Negro History Week (which later blossomed into Black History Month), he was also the principal of Lena's school, Dunbar High School in Washington, DC. While it is unclear how much they interacted, Lena remembered him well when she gave her oral history interview at seventy-seven years old.[6] Dr. Woodson and Lena's father likely influenced her college choice. After years of hard work and study, Lena was awarded the distinction of being named valedictorian of her 1918 class. Given Lena's credentials, people expected her to go to an Ivy League college. But she didn't want this. She wanted to attend a university that would strengthen her connection to the black community. Her father's alma mater seemed just the place to do that.

Lena experienced the stigma around attending historically black colleges and universities (HBCUs), which many students still experience today. Many of my friends who attended HBCUs as undergraduates tell me they are still asked by white peers to justify their decisions—even classmates at top medical schools react to HBCU grads with surprise, confusion, and, sometimes, suspicion. The absurd implication is that an HBCU education is subpar, that a person who attended one could never make it as far as they might have with a degree from a predominantly white institution (PWI). Obviously, that didn't occur in Lena's case. She had learned from her father's experience that she could thrive in an environment committed to black excellence. She attended Howard, instead of a PWI that held more prestige in certain spaces. When people questioned her choice, she said simply, "I'm going to stay and be educated at Howard University. I expect to devote my life to the development of my own people, and I'd rather live with them, and study with them at Howard."[7]

Dr. Lena Edwards had earned both her undergraduate and medical degrees from Howard University by 1924, six years after she graduated from high school. While at Howard, she became a member of Delta Sigma Theta Sorority, the country's second oldest historically black sorority. Following graduation, she started her internship at Howard's Freedmen's Hospital, joining the hospital the same year as Dr. Dorothy Ferebee. Notably, Dr. Edwards didn't seem to face the same challenges in finding an internship program that Dr. Ferebee did. Having attended a medical school affiliated with one of the few internship programs in the country that happily welcomed black physicians, Dr. Edwards easily transitioned from medical school to internship without having to face professors or residency admissions committees that wanted to deter her from her path.

For Dr. Edwards, medical school was more than just a space where she worked hard to reach her career goals. It was also the place where she met the love of her life: Keith Madison, a classmate. How did their love blossom? Did they meet on the first day of school and feel a spark that never seemed to wane? Did they start off as friends? Maybe they first became study buddies, just trying to make it through the grueling task of learning so much material, but one day their mounting feelings for each other could no longer be held back? I don't know. She didn't speak about it in her interviews. But I do know that having a decent number of black students in their medical school class allowed them to find each other and grow their relationship.

For Drs. Crumpler, Chinn, Ferebee, and any other black women physicians who entered medical school in the later nineteenth and early twentieth centuries, attending a predominantly white medical school meant they would be the only black student or one of a few black students in their classes. Many of these women were in their early to mid-twenties while in medical school, which is also the time when many would most likely find a partner. If they thought they could find their partner in school, something that was commonplace for their white counterparts, they were likely disappointed by their options. Just as white medical schools limited the number of women admitted every year, the schools set a very low quota for black students. If a black woman wasn't the only black person at her predominantly white medical school, the entering black class oftentimes looked like Dr. Chinn's: three black men and

May. Sadly, while the number of black male matriculants was higher than the number of black female matriculants in the early twentieth century, the overall graduation rate for black students was lower than that of white students, due to reduced financial support coupled with discrimination from many of their white medical professors. Whether it be black women or black men who were not able to graduate, the final graduation numbers for black students overall could be drastically lower than the number of black students who started. In Dr. Chinn's case, she and only one black man were able to complete their studies at New York University Medical College in 1926. With such a dismal number of black students in these predominantly white medical classes, it was rare for a romantic connection to develop between two black medical students.

Social stigma and legal battles likely blocked these women from considering interracial romance. As law professor Reginald Oh argues, racial segregation in schools was also a means of regulating gender relations between the two races—limiting or completely restricting the number of black students at a predominantly white school helped prevent interracial relationships.[8] The accuracy of this argument is easily seen today. Throughout my experience in higher education, I have met countless white people who said they never met a black person until they went to college. Due to historical redlining, coupled with people's personal preferences to live in communities with those who share their experiences, many neighborhoods have a predominantly white or black population—or a population made up predominantly of recent immigrants with similar ethnicities. Schools play a key role in how children and young adults form relationships with people from different backgrounds. Of the countless people I know who have had interracial relationships, the vast majority met their partners at school. If schools were still racially segregated, there would be many fewer interracial relationships today.

The black women who attended PWIs in the 1920s were some of the first black women to enter these medical school halls. In a space that disdained the presence of both black people and women, they were especially ostracized. White men viewed black women as another threat to their dominance within medicine. This made it difficult for black women to develop positive relationships with their white male class-mates. Dr. Chinn's experience with white male colleagues who wouldn't even acknowledge her presence in public is evidence of this.[9] If these white men couldn't even see these black women as worthy of respect, how could they view them as romantic prospects, to be loved and cher-ished? With the maltreatment that these black women endured from countless white men, as well as white women, it is unlikely that many of them saw white men or women as people they could imagine falling in love with. And when countless social barriers weren't enough to pre-vent a romantic connection between a black woman and a white man, law did the job. From 1860, when the first black woman started medical school, to June 12, 1967, when the *Loving v. Virginia* Supreme Court case was decided in favor of Mildred and Richard Loving, interracial mar-riage was illegal in much of the United States.

For the black women who attended PWIs, this likely delayed or de-railed their search for partners, which could also have prevented them from having kids. This is a perilous situation that many black women medical students find themselves in today. I know a number of black women doctors who were unable to have children as a result. Luckily for Dr. Lena Edwards, she found her husband at Howard, so she steamed ahead full force with shaping her professional and personal life in the way she wanted.

Following her internship at Howard's Freedmen's Hospital, Dr. Lena Edwards and Dr. Keith Madison moved to Jersey City, New Jersey, where the couple simultaneously opened a joint medical practice and started a family. Dr. Lena Edwards wanted children just as much as she wanted a career in medicine. She saw the two as intertwined: "I had an idea that so many children come from poor families, that a person who has had opportunities in education and a chance to make a decent living should have a whole lot of children, so that they could enjoy the best things in life."[10] And Dr. Lena Edwards did just that. Within a fourteen-year period, she had six children, all while maintaining her clinical practice.

She had her first child, Marie, two months after she started her medical practice. Marie followed in her parents' footsteps and became a physician. She graduated from Weill Cornell Medical College in 1951, becoming the first African American woman to earn her medical degree from this school.[11] Five months after Marie was born, Dr. Edwards became pregnant with her second child, Edward. He also became a physician after studying at Howard University College of Medicine, like his parents. Three years later, she had her third child, Genevieve, who earned bachelor's and master's degrees, focused on psychiatric sociology. Her fourth child, Thomas, became the chaplain of the Newman Center at Howard University. Her fifth child, John, was born in 1938 and became an aerospace engineer with NASA in Washington, DC. Her sixth child, Paul, was born in 1939 and became a high school teacher in New Jersey after earning his bachelor's degree. The immense success of the children, who grew up before and during the civil rights era, speaks to the impact these black physician parents had in helping their children navigate the hatred-laced landmines that served to decimate the success of many other black children at the time.

While Dr. Edwards was helping her children overcome obstacles in their professional lives, she continued to face challenges of her own. In 1931, the year after she had her third child, she was appointed to the staff of the Margaret Hague Maternity Hospital in Jersey City. Over the next few years, she saw assistant attending physicians and clinical attending physicians laid off if they did not have their board qualifications, which a physician can acquire only through the completion of a residency program.

Dr. Edwards saw these layoffs as a job opportunity for herself. While she had done an internship year at Howard, she had not completed a full residency program, which involves several years of postgraduate clinical training. She submitted her residency application to the Margaret Hague Maternity Hospital in 1936. Having already worked at the hospital for five years, she was confident about her chance of being accepted; the other doctors knew her personally, and they knew she was a talented and hardworking physician. So when she received their decision on her residency application, she was shocked. Rejection. Struggling to understand, she inquired into their rationale. Decades later, she hadn't forgotten the response from the hospital's chief of staff. She recalled: "I was told that I had two handicaps. First, I was a woman and that was worse than being a Negro."[12]

This was a punch to the gut. She had been sheltered from this level of prejudice at Howard. While the experience might have brought her down, she mirrored her father's resilience and got right back up. She prepared her residency application for the next cycle, adding to her résumé a year of experience from the very hospital where she sought residency training. Once again, she was rejected. She had weathered repudiation of qualities central to her personhood for eight years in a row. But she refused to give up. Finally, in her ninth consecutive year of applying to Margaret Hague's residency program, she was accepted. Dr. Lena Edwards completed the residency program and passed the qualifying exams, making her one of the first African American women to be a National Board-certified obstetrician-gynecologists in the US.[13] She used these credentials to secure a position as a gynecologist in the hospital's surgical department.

These credentials also allowed Dr. Edwards to reach for another rung of her career ladder: membership in the International College of Surgeons. As she researched the application process and those who were involved, she found out that the physician responsible for recommendations to the society didn't believe that women should be in medicine. Exhausted from tiptoeing around other people's prejudices, Lena was direct with this physician: "I went to him and told him I was applying, and I didn't expect him to refuse me, unless he had some real good excuse of lack of good quality in my work. 'So, I'm not going to wait until you blackball me, I'm telling you now—don't blackball me.' And I got in."[14]

Throughout her career, Dr. Edwards had to fight for her right to be in medicine. She had to be her own champion and cheerleader when she was surrounded by colleagues and superiors who sought to bring her down. Her advice to those in similar situations is to "go after what you want, and you have to go at it with determination and proficiency. When you get there, you have to be the best. And this has been the secret of my success, if I have any."[15] This is a mindset that many African Americans, in the past and present, have adopted as the primary tool for success in a society where they experience countless disadvantages due to their identity. Research studies are now exhibiting a truth African Americans have known for generations: If we have the same qualifications as a white person, that white person will usually be chosen over us for the opportunity.[16] The only way to combat this discrimination is to strive to be our best and, if we have the chance, work to change the system. The old adage, that black people have to work twice as hard to attain the same goals as white men, was on clear display once again.

Unfortunately, this strategy doesn't always work out. An aspiring black woman physician living in the South in the 1920s couldn't train at a southern PWI medical school, regardless of how talented she was or how hard she worked. Impenetrable institutional and social barriers made it impossible. Therefore, most early black women physicians trained in the Northeast. It was where opportunities for this demographic were concentrated. In Dr. Edwards's case, determination and proficiency transformed the small window of opportunity that she was given—a low-level job at a hospital—into a door that she could push open, allowing her to achieve much more. It allowed her to have a significant impact at Margaret Hague Maternity Hospital. She reached the point of managing 360 maternity cases and performing a hundred operations in a year. A pliable environment was necessary, but not sufficient, for Dr. Edwards's success.

While managing a high caseload, Dr. Edwards made sure her clinical practice was rooted in the humanity of medicine, an area in which many of her colleagues needed to improve substantially. Dr. Edwards recalled how the prestige of her hospital drew patients and medical students from all over the world for treatment and clinical training, respectively. There were times when international patients who spoke English as a second language struggled to communicate with their care team; many of the physicians in the practice responded to these patients with laughter. They really thought it was funny that vulnerable pregnant women in need of medical care couldn't even express whether they were experiencing excruciating pain in their enlarged bellies, or even if pain was present, due to the language barrier. Thankfully, Dr. Edwards did not take this stance. She had studied German, French, and Spanish when she was younger, and she used those skills to help bridge the cultural gap. Just by taking the time to sit down with the women and speak to them to the best of her ability, Dr. Edwards made medicine more accessible for people right in her neighborhood.

Language can be an impervious barrier, especially in a high-stress clinical setting. Dr. Edwards's respectful and intentional approach to such a challenge caught the attention of budding medical students who were still shaping their identities and clinical approach as future physicians. A young man that Dr. Edwards referred to as Evans was a medical student from Howard and the child of one of Dr. Edwards's high school friends. Evans witnessed her empathy in practice and shared with her the impact that she was having on his training: "You know, you're teaching us something about the humanity of medicine, and we're not getting it in school."

Flattered, but not too surprised, Dr. Edwards responded, "I know you're not. When I went through, we got it. But now everything is rush, rush, rush … People forget what I was first told when I was in medical school: 'When a patient walks into your office, watch him from the time he walks in your office to the time he walks out. Listen to everything he says. Let him sit comfortably in the office and tell you what he wants to tell you.'"[17]

Medicine was evolving at breakneck speed. As technology and research were advancing, some physicians were becoming more enmeshed with the science of medicine while losing sight of its art. You can't create a formula for how to interact with each patient. They're all different. It takes empathy and a bit of intuition to figure out how to interact with individuals. While it's difficult to become skillful at this art, it is essential that doctors work on the skill in order to provide adequate care to their patients. Dr. Edwards realized that she might be able to help change the new culture by returning to Howard to teach at the medical school. Inspired by the prospect of helping medical students become better doctors, and feeling freed by the fact that all her children had grown up and moved out of the house, Dr. Edwards moved back to DC in 1954 to teach medical humanities as an instructor at Howard University College of Medicine.

After six years of teaching, Dr. Edwards realized that she might want to retire soon. Before ending her medical career, she wanted to participate in a Christian mission trip, which she had been dreaming of doing for years. In 1960, she finally took the leap. She resigned from her lecturer post at Howard and moved to Hereford, Texas, to join the St. Joseph's Mission. She felt particularly compelled to join this mission because it served Mexican migrant farmworkers who played a crucial role in putting food on many Americans' tables, and yet were "treated worse than their cattle" in American society.[18] The mission sought to provide medical care for a community that had been deprived of this resource.

When Dr. Edwards joined the team at a hospital in Hereford she seemed to be the only woman on staff. It was quite unusual for a black woman to be able to attain a position at a hospital in the Jim Crow South that had previously employed only male physicians (likely white male physicians), but she was the only certified obstetrician-gynecologist within fifty miles.[19] Any prejudice was easily outweighed by the dire need for her expertise. When she joined the team, the hospital was in the process of certification. It needed a qualified ob-gyn to smooth the process. Aware of the hospital's predicament, Dr. Edwards leveraged its need when negotiating her position. She was able to acquire full privileges to practice at the hospital as an attending physician, allowing her to build a clientele list that she could use as she prepared to build a maternity clinic nearby. She was in awe once she realized how much she had accomplished. "Me. Deep in the heart of Texas. A black woman. A doctor."[20] She knew how difficult it was to gain any leadership position in the northern hospitals. The fact that she had garnered so much influence in the Jim Crow South was that much more remarkable. She had found a way to navigate the system, to leverage the power that she had and create her own opportunities.

Within two years, Dr. Edwards and her team had built a ten-bed maternity clinic. She also helped remodel an old, dilapidated clinic at a labor camp into a twenty-five-bed clinic dedicated to maternity care. Maintaining her conviction from her time at Howard to live and grow with the people she served, Dr. Edwards chose to live alongside the migrant workers on the labor camp grounds. Each morning, when the air was still crisp, but before the sun had peeked into the sky, Dr. Edwards would awaken for her house calls. She knew that the workers would be making tortillas by five in the morning, before they headed to work, so she would meet them for home visits before their breakfast had time to settle in their stomachs.

By spending so much time with the migrant workers, she had a chance to get to know them on a level deeper than their physical ailments. She got to know five young women who, although they worked as migrant workers, were truly passionate about medicine. Leveraging her leadership position at the clinic, she recruited some nurses from Saint Mary's School in Minneapolis to teach the migrant women how to become nurses' aides. One of the women loved the medical field so much that she studied to become a licensed vocational nurse. Still, she wanted to reach higher. She wanted to go to school to become a registered nurse, but she didn't earn enough money at the labor camp to pay for tuition. Dr. Edwards felt that she had a responsibility to use the privilege she had been afforded to help others, so she paid this young woman's tuition, allowing her to use her inherent talents and ambition to serve her community.

At the beginning of Dr. Edwards's time in Hereford, the workers didn't understand her generosity. Decades later, she still remembered the day when a young woman approached her and declared, "You know, my people can't understand you."

"Don't they like me?"

"Well, yes, but they wonder what's in it for you. That you're doing so much for us."[21]

Dr. Edwards understood their concerns. Many of the migrant workers were immigrants from Mexico. As an African American, Dr. Edwards could relate to their experience of oppression in the US. After living through so much hardship inflicted by those in power, it becomes difficult to trust the intentions of a newcomer who isn't connected to the community. Some are charitable out of ulterior motives—there is something "in it" for them. But this wasn't the case for Dr. Edwards. She was driven to do the work out of love for people and her passion for caring for underserved communities. With time, her pure intentions became clear to the workers. She just wanted to offer support to people from vulnerable communities. Although she was a trained obstetrician, she also practiced general medicine, to serve more of the workers. While at the labor camp, Dr. Edwards delivered some 320 babies and cared for more than 500 families.

After Dr. Edwards had been working in Texas for a few years, people started to take notice of her work. One day, her telephone rang. It was Gerri Major, associate editor of *Ebony* magazine, on the phone from Chicago. Since 1945, *Ebony* has been committed to highlighting the accomplishments of black Americans, and it is still active and influential today. The magazine believed Dr. Edwards's story was worth spotlighting, so Major went to Texas and spent four days with Dr. Edwards, learning about the doctor's efforts and taking photos of her working. In February 1962, *Ebony* published an extensive article detailing Dr. Lena Edwards's mission work, accompanied by multiple action photos, their vivid colors bringing her work to life. The same issue highlighted an extravagant party in honor of the daughter of Nat King Cole, world-renowned singer and jazz pianist. The party boasted many prominent guests, including then president John F. Kennedy. When the president was leafing through the *Ebony* issue, he came across the article on Dr. Edwards.

Dr. Edwards believed it was through this article that President Kennedy became aware of her work and subsequently directed Arthur Goldberg, secretary of labor at the time and later associate justice of the Supreme Court, to contact her. Soon after the publication of the *Ebony* issue, Goldberg sent Dr. Edwards a letter inviting her to join the Advisory Council on Employment Security. She served on that committee, and on the National Advisory Committee for Manpower Development and Training, for seven years.[22] Like her role in Texas, she used her position of power to advocate for the less fortunate. She made efforts to improve the situation of many African Americans in the US by helping them find jobs. Dr. Edwards subscribed to the old proverb: "Give a man a fish, and you feed him for a day. Teach a man to fish, and you feed him for a lifetime."

• • •

D r. Edwards received numerous awards for her service, most notably the Presidential Medal of Freedom, the highest civilian award in the United States. President Kennedy nominated Dr. Lena Edwards for the award in 1963. Unfortunately, he was not able to present her with the award; President Lyndon B. Johnson did the honors. In 1964, Dr. Edwards was invited to the White House, along with all the other Presidential Medal of Freedom awardees.

Without hesitation, Dr. Edwards brought her family to the White House to receive the award with her, but she was surprised to find that none of the other awardees had done the same. Still, her family's presence made the event even more memorable. As President Johnson walked through the crowd to greet the awardees and their guests, he stopped before Dr. Edwards's two-year-old grandson, Little Joe. This black boy stood no more than three feet tall and had his hand in the palm of his mom's hand. President Johnson bent down to pick the little boy up and gave him a hug. Immediately, a photographer snapped a photo. A few months later, Little Joe and his mother were surprised to receive a package from the president. When they tore off the wrapping paper, a photo of Little Joe's smiling face as he hugged the president beamed back at them. The framed photo has been a cherished memento for the family ever since.

I magine being the child of a mother who prevailed in the face of so much opposition. How much strength would arise inside of you after witnessing her exhibit such intractable persistence? For Marie, watching her mother's journey through the years helped her develop her own impenetrable strength, which shielded her against the prejudice that she faced along her own journey into medicine. Marie attended Fordham University in the Bronx, New York, in the early 1940s. When she was enrolled, female students were treated like second-class citizens. She experienced more than just disdainful remarks from sexist professors at Fordham, where, as at many other male-dominated universities, prejudice was institutionalized. Female students weren't even allowed on campus during the week; they could attend only on weekends. But Marie refused to let this mistreatment impact her. She graduated from Fordham summa cum laude and then matriculated at Weill Cornell Medical College in 1945, the same year that her mom was finally admitted into the residency program at the Margaret Hague Maternity Hospital.

While in medical school, she met Victor Metoyer Jr., an African American architectural draftsman from Omaha, Nebraska, who was stationed in New York City for World War II.[23] They quickly fell in love and got married, deciding to start a family soon after. Marie gave birth to two children while in medical school. Many women would have been intimidated by the prospect of having children during such a demanding stage of their training. But Marie knew that her mother had children in the early stages of her career, so she could look to her for guidance and support.

If balancing medical school and a family weren't difficult enough, Marie had to contend with professors who tried to tear her down. Many men were drafted into the war, leaving numerous medical school spots open. While many of the male medical school admissions officers would've liked to maintain the restrictions on the number of women entering a given class, their sexism was overridden by their capitalistic drive. Someone needed to pay the medical school fees. In such dire circumstances as a world war, they begrudgingly allowed women to fill that role.

Still, the professors didn't want to let up; many openly complained about the increasing numbers of women who had been enrolling in medical schools since the start of the war. They couldn't wait for the fighting to end so that men could dominate the medical field once more. Some of the professors even chided the women students, proclaiming that it was a waste to educate the female medical students because they would just drop out as soon as they got married and became pregnant. Marie felt targeted, but she would not fold. She persisted, like her mother. Dr. Marie Metoyer graduated in 1951 from Weill Cornell, not only as one of a handful of women in her class but as the first African American female graduate in its history.[24]

The newly minted Dr. Metoyer's next steps were also influenced by her mother. Dr. Edwards had grown tired of the segmentation of medicine. Heart pain? Go to one doctor. Digestive issues? Go to another. With so many medical specialties, Dr. Edwards felt that many doctors were losing sight of the whole picture. This could cause patients with complex illnesses to bounce between multiple medical providers without the treatment they needed, because the specialized physicians weren't seeing the ways that different symptoms were connected. This wasn't necessarily their fault. The separation of medical specialties lends itself to the segmentation of the body in the minds of doctors and patients alike. A patient may go to their gastroenterologist, a doctor who specializes in the digestive system, to check on their gallstones. With so much focus on their gallbladder and bile duct, they may forget the recurrent bouts of itching that began the week before. But itching can be a sign that the flow of bile in the biliary tract is obstructed by gallstones, which can be life threatening.

Dr. Edwards told her daughter that "in order to be a good doctor, you have to know the whole body from the gray hairs to ingrown toenails."[25] Dr. Metoyer took her mother's advice and practiced as a family doctor for fifteen years. She initially joined her parents to run the family medical practice in Jersey City, practicing obstetrics and gynecology alongside her mother. She moved next door to her parents and continued to grow her own family. When Dr. Edwards was at Howard University in DC, or at the labor camps in Hereford, Texas, Dr. Metoyer oversaw the business.

This was a family legacy. Marie's grandfather inspired her mother to go into medicine. Against the will of many white men in medicine, Dr. Lena Edwards made it through, demonstrating to her children that they could defy the odds and be great, when societal norms and even laws tried to say that they could not.

Dr. Marie Metoyer continued to chart new territory like her mother. Soon after Dr. Edwards returned to Jersey City and the family practice, in 1968, Dr. Metoyer moved to Vermont, although only briefly. Caring for five children and a busy family medicine practice had become tiring. She wanted something new. And she had felt inspired by President John

F. Kennedy's words on the importance of community mental health. Dr. Metoyer completed a psychiatry residency at the University of Vermont from 1968 to 1972, then completed a fellowship in community and child psychiatry. From 1972 to 1981, she was the only psychiatrist practicing in Vermont's Northeast Kingdom region, one of the most rural areas of the state.[26]

Once her children were all grown up and out of the house, Dr. Metoyer and her husband, Victor, moved to Manchester, New Hampshire. She practiced medicine there, becoming New Hampshire's first African American female psychiatrist, until she retired at seventy. She was also one of the first African Americans to practice psychiatry in Vermont.[27] In 2012, US senator Jeanne Shaheen of New Hampshire honored Dr. Metoyer for her service to the people of New Hampshire. Sadly, Dr. Marie Metoyer passed away on March 17, 2020.

Dr. Edwards began her journey as a physician due to the influence of her father, a dentist. He served as a role model, teaching her the necessary steps to be successful in the healthcare field. She passed this gift down to her children and her children's children. Dr. Edwards was the first in her family to become a doctor; now the number of doctors in her family tree has reached twenty-nine.[28] This is the legacy of a black family who had the support and resources to actually achieve their dreams. What this woman modeled was not just persistence and dedication, however; her gift was service to community—and not just her own, but communities of people who had been oppressed and marginalized, and who richly deserved support. That she was able to give so much of herself is a remarkable achievement.

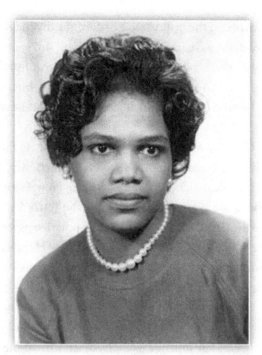

Dr. Edith Irby Jones

CHAPTER 5

FINDING FULFILLMENT IN GIVING BACK

B orn on December 23, 1927, to Robert Irby, a sharecropper, and his wife, Mattie Buice Irby, Edith Irby grew up near Conway, Arkansas. To Edith, it seemed her father did well for himself. He had a Model T Ford, a buggy, a wagon, and a horse. After church on Sundays, he would take the family in his Ford to a pump where they would collect fresh water to bring home.

Edith looked up to her father, and she remembered learning one of life's greatest lessons from him one Sunday, when she was just seven. She recounted the experience in a 2006 interview. Seated on a bench with a clear view of the front of their small church, young Edith watched as parishioners placed their tithes on a wooden table in the front of the room. Dressed in a stiff, white organdy dress with a patent-leather pocketbook at her side, she thought of the pennies she held in her purse.

As if reading her mind, Edith's father said, "Edith, you should go up and put your money on the table."

"No, no, Papa. I want to keep my money."

"No. You go up and you put it on, because when you give, you get back much more than you give. So, you give that in order that you can receive more."

Excited by the prospect of more pennies jingling in her pocketbook, Edith hurried off the bench and placed her money on the table. Then, she stood there and waited.

Eventually, Edith's father went up to her and said, "Edith, why don't you come back to sit down?"

She replied, "Papa, I was waiting for them to give me my money back, and more."

Realizing her misinterpretation of his words, Edith's father smiled as he explained, "Edith, you don't get it back all at that time, but when you give, you do get back in multiples, but it may not come back at the same time nor from the same source that you give it."[1] This message stuck with Edith and became her philosophy in life.

After church that day, Edith's mother and father went horseback riding. The outing was cut short when Robert was bucked from his horse. Unconscious, he was brought into the front room of their shotgun house, where someone tried to resuscitate him, blowing into his mouth and pumping his chest. This went on for some time to no avail. Robert Irby died.

Recalling that crushing day, Edith explained: "For that day, life, I would say, began. . . . That was when I grew up."[2] Edith watched as her mother wailed, recognizing how lost she must have felt. She wanted to help in some way, take on some responsibility. But the burden was far too great for a seven-year-old child who, even when she wanted to help her mother, was mourning a significant loss of her own for the first time.

On top of the grief, the crushing weight of supporting a family was stacked on Mattie Irby's shoulders. Not only was she left with twelve-year-old Juanita, nine-year-old Robert Jr., and seven-year-old Edith, but she was also pregnant with the family's fourth child. Mattie had an eighth-grade education and had learned only how to tend a home and raise her children. The family's modest income suddenly vanished, and destitution rushed in to take its place.

After Robert's death, Mattie learned that he had borrowed twenty-five dollars from the owner of the farm to make the crop for that year. Because Mattie was unable to find a job, she had no way of repaying the debt. The family was evicted, and the farmer seized all of Robert's property as compensation for the unpaid debt. Overnight, everything had been taken: the Model T, the buggy, the family's share of the crop, and their home.

Suddenly without a husband, a home, or a means to provide for her family, Mattie felt the new burden intensely. She desperately needed help caring for her three young children, plus a fourth growing inside her. She moved the family to Conway, Arkansas, to live with her father.

He promised the emotional and financial support their little family so desperately needed, but within weeks of their arrival, he passed away of natural causes. Faced with another loss so soon after Robert's death, Mattie could've been lost to her misery. The only thing that kept her afloat was an unflagging determination to care for her children. While they did suffer, the Irbys weathered the difficult times as a family, and they were closer for it. Unfortunately, the storm had not yet passed.

Only a few weeks after Mattie's father died, a typhoid outbreak spread throughout Conway. When rose-colored spots began appearing on Juanita and Robert Jr., Mattie knew something was wrong; the devastating illness had reached the Irby home. But Mattie refused to let her older daughter and son die without a fight. With barely enough money coming in just to get by and feed the family, she didn't have the means to pay for intensive medical care for her children. Instead, Mattie took her children's care into her own hands, enlisting the help of her youngest, Edith. At just seven, Edith took on bedside tasks gruesome enough to make an adult queasy. She tended to bedridden Juanita and Robert Jr. in the worst throes of typhoid, all while grieving both her father and grandfather.

As Edith and her mother struggled to care for their sick family, Edith noticed a white man in a white coat making regular visits to her neighbors. He had to be a doctor. Her older siblings were in a dire condition. Why wouldn't the doctor come to help them? Their medical condition wasn't much different from their neighbors'. What was? Well, she knew her neighbors' houses were bigger than hers. The kids had nicer clothes. Some of her neighbors even had cars.

Edith was young, but she wasn't naïve. After reflecting on their divergent lifestyles, she knew that the disparity in access to healthcare had to be related to money. As the children's health deteriorated, Mattie was able to scrape together enough money to afford a single visit by a doctor. She willingly sacrificed key essentials, like food, in an attempt to get her babies the care they needed. But this wasn't enough.

Juanita had numerous bouts of bloody diarrhea. She was hemorrhaging in some part of her intestines. Once the family noticed this, someone ran to the doctor's office and begged for his help. But he was busy. He had already made an appointment with one of Edith's neighbors. Their money commanded more attention than a girl experiencing a medical emergency did.

Edith watched helplessly while her older sister's life slipped away, and her conviction cemented as her heart broke from yet another loss of someone she loved dearly. "It was then that I vowed that my sister would not have died if she could have paid for having [the doctor] to come to see her as . . . often as he had gone to see the other children. And it was then that I resolved that I was going to be a doctor. . . . But I was gonna be a different kind of doctor. I was gonna be [the] doctor in which money wasn't gonna make any difference with me—that I was gonna particular see that those who did not have money—those who were less fortunate—would get the kind of care that they needed—that I was gonna do it as much as I could do it, and I was gonna instill into others that they must do it, too."[3]

After Mattie recovered from the deep sorrow of her loss, she began to focus on the future of her surviving children: Robert Jr. recovered from typhoid, Edith miraculously never caught the fever, and Mattie's youngest son, Louis, was born shortly after Juanita's death. Mattie didn't want her children just to survive, she wanted them to thrive, and she believed the best path to a good life was through a strong education. Not convinced that Conway could provide that for her children, she moved the family to Hot Springs, Arkansas.

Although racial segregation was the norm in the South, the Irby family entered a racially integrated community in Hot Springs. They had white neighbors, and Edith quickly befriended two girls her age. They played together without issue in the neighborhood. When they went to separate schools, Edith didn't realize that this separation was due partially to laws preventing the mixing of black and white children in southern schools. She chalked up the difference in schooling to finances: her family was still struggling, so she figured that her mother was not able to pay for the nicer school that her friends attended.

While the southern black schools, with their ragged books and underpaid teachers, rarely had the resources to set their students on promising career paths, Edith's circumstances allowed her to sidestep this barrier. Her mother became a maid for a young couple, Dr. Ellis and his wife, who had an eighteen-month-old son. When Mattie needed to work and watch her daughter, she brought Edith to the Ellises' house. She was only ten, and her youth caused the Ellis family to see past traditional color lines. As had been the case for May Chinn with the Tiffany family, Edith was treated like another child in the Ellis household. The family encouraged her, saying, "Stay in school. Be whatever you want to be. You can do it."[4] They also gave her access to the house library. Edith quickly developed a love for literature, devouring any book that she could put her hands on.

This intellectual drive translated to natural success in her studies. Edith's strong academic performance in high school marked her as a child to watch in Hot Springs. She was a black girl so smart that even the shackles of the Jim Crow South could not keep her from her goals. The neighborhood families were aware of Mattie's financial hardships, so they often stepped up to help Edith and her brothers. When Edith qualified to give speeches at various events, the clubs and the local church hosting the events raised money to buy her a proper outfit. Some people even sponsored her trips to church conferences outside of Hot Springs. It seemed like the whole community rallied around this bright young student, but strangers weren't the only ones making sacrifices for Edith.

One Easter, Edith was chosen to give the leading speech for a Sunday school church convention, but because she didn't have anything to wear, she was nervous she'd have to turn it down. When Edith told her mother about her predicament, Mattie went to her own closet and without so much as a second thought, pulled out her only nice dress and took down Edith's measurements. She spent the entire night resewing the dress to fit her daughter, an act typical of the personal sacrifices Mattie would make when it meant a greater chance of success for her children. In that dress, Edith remembered, she had felt confident and beautiful while giving her speech. Of course, without anything to wear herself, Mattie was unable to attend the service to watch Edith speak. She waited to hear it all retold when Edith got home.

The unwavering support that Edith received from her mother and the broader community emboldened her to believe that neither financial nor racial constraints would impede her success. When she graduated from high school in 1944, Edith took this mindset into the next stage of her life.

Eager to continue her education, Edith applied to and was accepted at Knoxville College in Tennessee. Still poor, her family didn't have enough money even to pay for school supplies. So, the summer before college, she left her home in Arkansas and moved in with her uncle and aunt on the South Side of Chicago, having heard that African Americans could find higher paying work in the North. She found a job as a typist and earned enough money to sustain herself over the summer, buy some school clothes, and move to Knoxville. After these expenses, Edith had just $60 to spare, not nearly enough to pay the $300 tuition at Knoxville College. Undeterred, Edith made her way back south anyway.

She arrived at Knoxville College with her registration forms and her $60. When it came time to register for classes, Edith joined a long line of students at the registrar's office. A voice from the office called out, "Those who have everything they need, get in this line. Let's see if we can't move it a little faster. And those who know they need something else, stand in the other line."

With only a fifth of tuition, Edith moved into the other line. With each step forward, the line shortened until finally Edith stood face-to-face with the registrar. "Young lady, what is it that you need?"

Holding her summer earnings in her hand, Edith said, "Tuition is $300, but I don't have but $60."

Bluntly, the registrar responded, "Well, I can't help you."

Undeterred, Edith asked, "Oh? Who can?"

"No one can help you here but the president."

Sensing a solution to her problem, Edith replied, "Where is he? May I see him?"

After walking down the hall, Edith was introduced to the president of the college, Dr. William Lloyd Imes. She didn't waste any time. "Dr. Imes, I'm Edith Irby. I want to enroll as a freshman, but I don't have all of the tuition."

Struck by her boldness, Dr. Imes asked, "How much do you have?"

"I have $60."

Shocked, he replied, "Tuition is $300."

Familiar with finding ways around financial constraints, Edith explained, "Yes, sir, I know. But I don't have $300. I don't have any place I can get $300, and I want to go to school at Knoxville College."

Because Knoxville was, and still is, a historically black college that supports black students in difficult circumstances, Dr. Imes tried to figure out how to accommodate Edith's situation. "Can you work?"

Seeing an opening, she said, "Sure, I can work. I can type. I can do most other things if I need to, but I need to go to college."

"Can you take shorthand too?"

"Yes, sir."

"Well, my secretary is sick today. Could you take a letter for me?"

Edith pounced on the opportunity, typing his letter quickly and handing it back to him.

Dr. Imes looked it over. He was so impressed that he hired Edith on the spot. "You can be my secretary's assistant secretary. We will see that you get your tuition and your other bills paid."[5]

Edith was over the moon to be pursuing her education. She immersed herself in all that college had to offer. She got involved in the student government and the debate team, became a cheerleader, and even played some basketball on the side. She also joined Delta Sigma Theta Sorority. Throughout her undergraduate years, Edith continued working as an assistant secretary in the president's office while moonlighting at the canteen and drugstore to make extra money that she sent back home to support Mattie and Louis, her younger brother. Even with all her extracurricular involvement, Edith's focus never wavered from her studies. Determined to obtain a good education, she triple-majored in chemistry, biology, and physics, earning a final transcript studded with As. Edith's strong academic performance distinguished her in the eyes of her instructors. A number of her professors, including the vice president of the college, wrote recommendations in support of her entry into medical school. It was clear that Edith had the intellectual and emotional capacity needed to succeed as a doctor. Her next step after graduation was to raise money to finance her medical education.

Edith returned to Chicago and to the company where she had previously been a typist. She was promoted to manager of personnel. During the days, she worked long hours to earn money for school. In the evenings, she took a clinical psychology course at Northwestern University to strengthen her medical school application. The high cost of applying to medical school quickly depleted any funds she was able to raise. The sixty dollars she had raised four years earlier for tuition at Knoxville College was a distant memory, dwarfed by the mounting cost of applying to twelve medical schools at a cost of five to ten dollars for each submission.

Edith hadn't let financial obstacles stand in the way of her dreams before, and she wasn't about to start now. She recalled the mindset that she held throughout her life: "If you're persistent—if you intend for it to happen, it will happen. I have no doubt that things that we fail in are the things that we are not persistent about enough to achieve."[6] Confident that this persistence would carry her through, she worked through one challenge at a time. The first step had been financing her medical school applications; she would worry about the cost of attendance once she got there.

After one long day of work, Edith had returned to her uncle's home when she received an unexpected phone call.

"This is *Time* magazine. I called to find out if you are going to accept your place at the University of Arkansas."

Shocked, Edith responded, "I have not been accepted yet."

"Yes, you have been." Eager to get the inside scoop on this historic decision, the reporter pressed: "But we want to know if you're going to—if you're going."

Without a second's hesitation, Edith declared, "Yes, I'm going."[7]

Edith graduated from Knoxville College in the spring of 1948, when racial segregation still permeated the education system in the Jim Crow South. If an African American from the South wanted to earn an undergraduate or professional degree, they usually had to attend one of the historically black colleges and universities, or an integrated school in the North. Never had a black person attended a predominantly white medical school in the South. Edith's decision to enroll at the University of Arkansas School of Medicine would make her the first.[8]

Before her acceptance at the University of Arkansas, she had already been accepted at the University of Chicago School of Medicine and Northwestern University Medical School. Once the news broke of her acceptance into a southern medical school, additional acceptance letters poured in. Northwestern and the University of Chicago even told her that if she went to the University of Arkansas for a few weeks and found the racial discrimination to be unbearable, she could transfer and the schools would give her a tutor to help her catch up. Despite these generous offers, Edith decided to stick with her initial decision to attend the University of Arkansas School of Medicine, which was only about an hour away from her home in Conway.

Edith had spent all the money she had earned in Chicago on her medical school applications and on the clinical psychology course at Northwestern. She didn't have any money left to pay for medical school. Still, she pushed forward with her plans.

Edith recalled, "All I wanted to do was go to medical school. . . . I had spent my whole life getting ready to go to medical school, and now I had a chance to go to medical school. . . . I had been accepted. . . . And nothing else made any difference. . . . Segregation didn't make any difference. Money didn't make any difference. Absolutely nothing made any difference. I had reached the point in life that I intended to get: accepted in medical school."[9]

As it had when she was in high school, Edith's Arkansas support system rallied around her. After paying the bus fare from Chicago back to Arkansas, Edith had only five dollars to her name. Tuition at the University of Arkansas was $500. When her community heard that Edith was struggling, it rallied to support her. After church, people passed the hat. Any change they could contribute, they did. Even the white mayor pitched in his support. Lack of money was just one of many hoops that black people had to jump through to make it to medical school. Edith was the first in the community to have made it over countless other barriers, from gaining access to college to convincing professors to recommend her for medical school. She had made it so far. Though many of the community members had financial struggles themselves, they were unwilling to let finances be the blockade that stopped Edith from achieving her destiny. Unfortunately, costs continue to block many aspiring black physicians to this day. With the cost of medical school skyrocketing from $500 to $400,000, it is no longer enough to pass the hat to help a promising low-income student attend medical school. Many students are instead forced to decide between taking on the crippling burden of loans, which could plague them for decades, or give up their dreams of becoming physicians.

Edith accepted her community's monetary contributions with immense gratitude and responsibility. "It was . . . I don't even know the word that I could say. . . . It was hometown support, but the feeling I had for it was, 'I have everybody behind me. I don't have any choice but to succeed. . . . They've put me here. I've got to succeed.' And it wasn't a white/black issue. It was—the whites were putting in. They were putting in as much as the blacks were."[10]

As Edith registered for class, she discovered that she needed $50 in addition to tuition, to pay for labs and incidentals. She had only a dollar or two left. But she remembered a friend who could help her. Edith had met Thad Williams, a graduate of Morehouse College, when both were undergraduates riding the segregated trains to and from school and home for school vacations. In the summertime, Williams worked for the *Arkansas State Press*, located in Little Rock, near Edith's medical school. When Williams had found out that Edith was accepted into the University of Arkansas, he told her that if she ever needed any help she should go to Daisy and L. C. Bates, who ran the *State Press*. In need of the last $50 to register for school, Edith did exactly this. She stopped in the middle of the registration process and took the bus down to the *State Press*.

Once at the office, Edith asked the nearest person, "Is Mr. or Mrs. Bates here?"

"I'm Daisy Bates. Can I help you?"

Not shy about her situation, Edith responded, "Mrs. Bates, I need $50. I'm trying to register to—"

"What? You need $50? Why do you need $50?"

"I'm trying to register in medical school. I'm Edith Mae Irby, and I need $50 more than the money I have to register."[11]

Recognizing Edith's name, Daisy gave Edith the $50 without another word. Every Saturday after their meeting, Daisy brought Edith $25 or $30 to pay for food, clothing, transportation, and other essentials. Daisy collected this money from the black professionals who congregated on Ninth Street near the *Press*. She would just walk out of the office and say, "Give me $5. Give me $10. This is for Edith Irby."[12]

Daisy and L. C. Bates also invited Edith into their home. Every weekend, the couple played poker, and when Edith was able to take a break from her studies she would go to play poker with them, instead of spending the weekends alone. During these games, she met many of Little Rock's black elite. She became known as a socialite and was invited to many parties, where she was introduced to the world of advocacy. The Bateses were heavily involved in the civil rights movement, and as Edith learned and became more involved herself, she was even invited to speak at various advocacy events.

One of the more significant events she attended was hosted by the National Association for the Advancement of Colored People (NAACP), in New Orleans. She was asked to give a speech at the event, alongside Thurgood Marshall, the lawyer who would successfully argue before the US Supreme Court in the *Brown v. Board of Education* case as the legal counsel for the NAACP and in 1967, become the first African American associate justice of the Supreme Court.

Because black people didn't typically ride airplanes in the 1940s, Thurgood Marshall picked up Edith from school in his black Cadillac and drove her from Little Rock to New Orleans. During the seven-hour ride, Thurgood probed Edith about her experience in medical school. First he asked about her overall well-being and academic performance. Then he broached the topic of finances.

"What do you do for money? Where is your money?"

Surprised, Edith had to consider how to answer. "I get enough."

Not convinced, Thurgood persisted, "Well, how do you get it?"

"People send it to me. They put dollars in envelopes, and Mrs. Bates brings me some. And some people put money on a card, you know, and paste it on the card so it doesn't juggle around it. They send me that. Maybe fifty cents at a time."

Edith felt she was doing okay; she had a lifetime's worth of experience stretching the spare change that came her way. She was just grateful for the goodwill. But Thurgood recognized that she was struggling. He declared, "That's no way to live."[13] After the conference, he went back home to Harlem, New York. He lived on 409 Edgecombe Avenue, where Dr. May Chinn was also living at the time, along with multiple leaders of the Harlem Renaissance.[14] Once he was home, Thurgood shared Edith's situation with Dr. William Montague Cobb, a physician-scientist and the first African American to earn a PhD in anthropology.[15] Dr. Cobb was also a civil rights activist committed to countering the negative impact racism had on communities of color. Dr. Cobb and Thurgood Marshall recognized how essential Edith's success was to increasing opportunities for the entire black community, so they worked together to ease Edith's journey. Eventually, they found a wealthy woman in New York who was willing to sponsor Edith's medical education. All Edith had to do was write down all her expenses: tuition, room and board, food, transportation, clothes. The total was $3,000 each year, which is worth approximately $35,000 today. Edith thought this amount was too large of a request. But her sponsor knew that Edith was worth investing in, so she sent Edith the entire amount without hesitation.

The comfort and stability that this arrangement granted Edith was threatened when she was struck by loss yet again. During Edith's second year of medical school, her mother, Mattie, died. As had happened when Edith lost family members when she was a child, she didn't have the luxury to just mourn. She had to think about her younger brother, fifteen-year-old Louis, who had just lost his sole caretaker. Suddenly, this responsibility fell on Edith. Would she drop out of medical school to take care of her brother, or abandon him to the foster system so that she could continue her medical education? Thankfully, she was spared from deciding between these impossible choices when Thurgood Marshall heard of her predicament. He stepped in and raised additional funds to keep Louis in boarding school. With this financial backing, Edith was able to stay in medical school while her brother continued his education in a stable environment.

Everyone watching Edith knew that she was making history, so they did whatever they could to help her on her journey. At the time, Edith didn't consider her role in the grand scheme of things. She was just a young person who wanted to go to medical school and become a doctor. Nothing else mattered to her. She didn't want to think about the politics of it all. She just wanted to pursue her dream.

Though the politics weren't important to Edith, her success was tied directly to them. She wasn't like the white students who could become physicians based on their intellect and their connections to influential people within medicine. She wasn't like the black students who were smart but were prevented from advancing into medicine because of racism. Edith had entered a new stratum as the first African American to attend a predominantly white medical school in the South. Unlike when Dr. Rebecca Lee Crumpler entered medical school in 1860, when Edith Irby broke the color line within the southern medical community eighty-eight years later, people thought it was an achievement worth remembering.

On Edith's first day of medical school, *Life* magazine shot a photo of the groundbreaking moment: Edith Irby, the first African American medical student to break into this exclusively white space. The photo shows Edith standing in a hallway as a few of her white male classmates look in her direction. She appears totally alienated in the space, but that wasn't the message she wanted to spread. She wanted to be just another medical student, not the token minority that everyone gawked at. Edith didn't see herself as the poster child for victims of racial dis-crimination and oppression. Because she was raised in the South with amicable white neighbors, she had learned how to navigate systemic racism while creating meaningful bonds with white members of the community. Edith maintained a similar balance when she became the first and only African American medical student at the University of Arkansas in 1948.

Soon after Edith matriculated, Dr. Henry Clay Chenault, dean of the University of Arkansas School of Medicine, called her into his office to tell her some difficult news. As Edith recounted, he said to her: "They say if I let you eat in the dining room with the whites, that they're gonna raise a stink. And I'm not going to let you eat with the help. So I'm going to give you separate quarters. You're gonna eat in the library in a special room that's gonna be set up for you, for you to have lunch. I hope you understand. I've got to stay here, and I want you to stay here."[16]

Dr. Chenault believed that his position at the medical school would be jeopardized if he let Edith eat with her classmates, so he used his power to protect himself. Edith accepted her situation, feeling like she had no other option. Reflecting on this instance of racial segregation in the South, she later declared, "That's the way it was."[17]

The school's staff felt badly for Edith. They tried to make the library a nice space for her. They covered the study desk, where she was meant to eat, with a white tablecloth, and they placed live flowers on the table each day. Once, Edith came to lunch to find a note that read, "We love you."[18]

Within a few days of matriculation, some of her classmates decided to bridge the gap between Edith and themselves. Jim Crow laws said that blacks and whites couldn't eat together in public, but Edith's setup made for a loophole in the restrictions. The library was considered a private space, so some of her fellow students felt comfortable eating with Edith there. Outside of lunch, too, Edith's classmates would join her in the section of the library where she was allowed to study.

The dining room and study areas weren't the only spaces where racist restrictions impacted Edith's access to campus amenities. She wasn't even allowed to use the women's bathroom. Because she was the first black student, the school didn't have a "blacks only" women's bathroom. The only student bathrooms on campus were for white men and white women. Again, it was Dr. Chenault who broke the news to her. "If they find out, they're gonna use everything they can to impede our progress. So I'm gonna give you a special toilet. We're not going to mark it, but it's yours. The help knows not to use it."[19]

What impact could this social isolation have had on her emotional well-being? Could being compelled to use areas of the school typically reserved for "the help" have made her feel more like a member of the staff than a member of the next generation of physicians?

———•—•—•———

I can attest to how lonely medical school can be. Oftentimes, I have lectures from eight in the morning to six in the evening with few breaks. The bulk of the material is new, so the rest of the night after class is spent trying to understand what I was taught during the day. Because I'm more productive studying alone, I'm forced to decide between being around other people and being productive during my packed schedule. Beginning this training during COVID-19 has made the social experience only more challenging. Most of my classes are virtual, so I spend most of the time studying in my apartment. When exams approach, I can go days without leaving my building.

The infrequent opportunities I have had to get together with my classmates have made a huge difference in my experience. Though these days the opportunities look like socially distanced picnics in the park, instead of lunch in the school dining room, I cherish the moments that I'm able to spend with fellow students. Social time, especially with my classmates who know exactly what I'm going through, keeps me energized and helps ward off burnout, an extremely common issue within medicine.

I can't imagine how I would react if the dean of my medical school told me that I had to eat in the library or in a "blacks only" section of the park, away from the rest of my classmates. Dr. Chenault may have been just the messenger, rather than someone who truly believed that Edith should be separated from her classmates. But for me, as someone who is still trying to find my footing within medicine, still trying to convince myself that I will become a doctor, the words and actions of the established physician leading my medical school would have defined my experience and sense of belonging. I imagine it would be nearly impossible to endure the grueling nature of medical school while also coping with a regional policy reinforced by the dean that demanded I be separated from the entirety of my class, other than the few classmates who defied the norms of the time to interact with the sole black student. Without even considering the financial and personal challenges Edith faced, her ability to complete medical school as the only student directly impacted by her school's segregation policies was an incredible feat.

Undeterred by the racial divide, Edith developed close friendships with some of her white classmates. One of her closest friends was a woman named Mary Arthur. Though different they may have looked— Edith with her curly dark-brown hair and almond-brown skin next to Mary's straight blond hair, blue eyes, and pale complexion—Edith felt like Mary could have been her sister. Because of their stark physical differences, the women knew to be careful when they were together, acutely aware of the social consequences of being seen spending time with someone of another race. When the women rode the bus together, they knew not to sit together. It could ignite violence from a white person intolerant of positive connection between members of the two races. Edith described the scenario of sitting together on the bus as "the worst thing we could do."[20] Aware of the signs instructing whites to sit in the front and blacks to sit in the back, they thought of a way to stay together on a technicality. They stood on the bus, instead of sitting. It didn't matter if most of the seats were empty. They remained standing.

While they thought standing would prevent unwanted attention, people took note of the amicable conversation and laughs that they shared with each other. No one said anything to them directly. Still, rumors spread. Mary's father was a well-known veterinarian for the state. When word got back to him that Mary was riding the bus with a black girl, something that could have brought harm to both women, he bought Mary a car. Despite the frightening truth that her friendship with Mary might provoke racist violence, Edith focused on the positive. She was glad that Mary got a car; now it was easier for them to get to school together.

No part of Edith's life went unmonitored. She even had to be careful of how late she studied with her classmates. When she rented her own apartment, she was excited to share the space with her friends. Given the intense workload of medical school, studying became a primary way for classmates to spend time together. During the more intense weeks, they would study until one or two in the morning. Edith's white classmates without cars were afraid to call cabs to pick them up from Edith's home. They worried that if someone took notice of their late-night interracial gathering, things could turn violent.[21]

On nights when Edith was able to finish studying earlier in the evening, she spent her free hours advocating for civil rights. Around seven in the evening, she would change out of her school clothes, put on a dressier outfit, and shrug off the stress of the school day. Then she would attend rallies at schools and churches, telling people that they didn't have to accept a life that was supposedly "separate but equal." They didn't have to accept the secondhand books with pages torn out of them, or with scribbles over the text, from the white children who had used the books before them and wanted to hinder the black children from learning the material. These separate resources were not equal. Edith discouraged protests, but through spreading the word, she emboldened others to speak up against racial injustice. She engaged in this advocacy work with lawyers Bob Booker, Floyd Davis, and Harold Flowers, who had all played key roles in desegregating the University of Arkansas School of Law the same year Edith started at the medical school.[22] Together, the four of them were known as the Freedom Four. They went all over Arkansas advocating for the end of Jim Crow laws.

This advocacy work could have gotten Edith in trouble with the medical school because she risked being accused of inciting social unrest. While becoming a physician was her ultimate dream, she was passionate enough about ending systemic racism in the South that she put her career on the line. Edith was able to navigate the Jim Crow South relatively unscathed, but she saw many African Americans suffering because of the systemic inequities. She knew her platform as the first black medical student in the South could help make a difference. "I was young and brave and fearless and felt that I had a cause for which to be concerned, and never really feared."[23] She kept up with her studies amid this socially active schedule by studying whenever she could. She would study in the car on the way to events, and sometimes she would even study at the event, when she wasn't busy giving a speech or talking to a community member.

As busy as she was professionally, Edith also found a way to maintain a personal life too. She met her husband, Dr. James B. Jones, during a summer break in medical school. He was the first African American to earn a PhD at the University of Washington in Seattle.[24] They immediately bonded over the shared struggle of being the first person to integrate a school. James loved and supported Edith through the personal and professional challenges she faced throughout this time. They married when Edith was a second-year medical student.[25]

Dr. Edith Irby Jones completed her medical training, graduating from the University of Arkansas School of Medicine in 1952, two years before the *Brown v. Board of Education* Supreme Court decision declared racially segregated public schools to be unconstitutional. She then began a pediatrics residency at a hospital in Hot Springs, Arkansas, making her the first African American to do so. Her relationship with the dean, Dr. Chenault, had strengthened throughout her years in medical school. When he retired from the medical school and started working at a urology, obstetrics, and gynecology clinic near Edith's hospital, she sought guidance and support from him and other physicians at the clinic. They taught her various techniques that she hadn't learned in her residency, such as how to work on gallbladders and treat appendicitis. She also worked for them as a medical consultant on difficult cases.

During her first year of residency, Edith got pregnant. She was aware of the challenges that black women faced when they gave birth, particularly in the segregated South, so she made special arrangements to deliver her baby at the hospital where she was a resident. Receiving medical care from physicians whom she knew personally was supposed to protect her from the maltreatment that many black patients received in the Jim Crow South. But when Edith's water broke and she was ready to give birth, she was forced to sit in the parking area outside of the hospital because the obstetric physician and his medical staff were not prepared to help Edith deliver her baby. The familiar Arkansas heat likely felt uncomfortable to Edith as her contractions grew closer together. She had learned about childbirth in her medical training, but the textbook descriptions and visual demonstrations were nothing compared to this new feeling inside her body. She needed to be admitted to the hospital as soon as possible. A cool hospital room could go a long way in easing her discomfort.

Her personal physician became agitated by the administrative difficulties at the hospital. He insisted that she go to a private hospital to give birth, even though it was for white patients only. While she was likely wary of going to an all-white hospital for medical care, her labor had progressed to a point where it was her only choice. She was carted off to the all-white hospital.

As the hours of labor passed, complications emerged. Maybe her delivery was prolonged, or her baby was in the breech position, his feet facing downward—which is dangerous in a vaginal delivery. Whatever the reason, the doctors decided it was necessary for Edith to have a C-section instead of the natural birth that she had hoped for. A C-section is a major surgery that requires postoperative care. It's associated with serious postoperative risks, such as intense pain, wound separation, infection, and even deep vein thrombosis, which can be deadly.[26] To prevent some of these negative outcomes, women are supposed to be monitored in the hospital for at least twelve hours after the procedure. The all-white hospital leaders were well aware of how important it is to watch a woman who has just undergone the surgery, but they refused to admit a black patient into one of its hospital rooms. It didn't matter if the patient was the first black physician to train in the South, or the highest-ranking black lawyer in the country. It didn't matter if refusing to admit the black patient could lead to their death. To allow a black patient to lie in a hospital bed in a room adjacent to a white patient's—they would never stoop that low.

Unwilling to taint its precious hospital with racial mixing, the facility administrators sent Edith home immediately after her surgery. She hadn't even reached the point of recovery where her husband could take her home himself. She was swooped up by an ambulance and dropped off at her house, where the only medical care she or her hours-old baby had access to was the care that she could provide herself. Her medical knowledge became useful when it was time to circumcise her son, Gary. While she was still recovering from her surgery, Edith taught her husband how to perform a circumcision. Using sterile surgical instruments from the hospital, he completed the procedure on his newborn son on the family's kitchen table.

Dr. Irby Jones wasn't new to the neglect of black people by the medical system. She had experienced it her whole life, though she had obviously hoped that her situation would improve once she joined the medical ranks. Sadly, this was not the case—at least not in the delivery room. Black women commonly receive worse care during child delivery, and they experience higher maternal and infant mortality rates. Even today, more than sixty years after Dr. Irby Jones's terrifying experience as a patient in the maternity ward, black women are three times more likely to die from pregnancy-related causes than white women are.[27] But if becoming a physician isn't enough to protect a black woman when she undergoes this popular medical procedure, what is?

I am all too familiar with the challenges black women experience while giving birth. Over and over, I have read the statistics about poorer health outcomes for black mothers and their babies. The horror stories from black women in the delivery room reverberate in my mind as I try to go to sleep. It seems that all too often, medical personnel do not believe the amount of pain these women are in, causing clinicians to miss key signs that the women are experiencing serious complications. High-profile stories, like that of tennis superstar Serena Williams, send chills down my spine. If one of the world's best-known athletes almost died after giving birth, how can I be confident that I will survive when that day comes for me?

My desire to become a physician was partially motivated by my desire to live, and to be able to protect myself, in moments when others would not, based solely on my race. If I were to have a child after my residency, I would certainly think that making plans to deliver my baby at the hospital where I worked would keep me safe. Dr. Irby Jones's experience shows me that this may not be the case. While she gave birth in an era when racial segregation of hospitals was still common, the perpetually high rates of maternal and infant mortality in black families indicates that there is still a problem. Researchers and advocates must continue trying to elucidate and correct the factors that contribute to this health disparity. Childbirth needs to be made safer for black women around the country. Our lives depend on it.

Thankfully, the doctor who encouraged Dr. Jones to go to the all-white hospital would not tolerate this medical injustice. After seeing how the hospital treated Dr. Irby Jones, he refused to treat any of his patients there, regardless of their race. Within a week, pressure from this white physician and others led to the closing of the hospital.[28]

After recovering from childbirth, Dr. Irby Jones returned to work in Hot Springs, where she remained for six years. Her husband was teaching in Pine Bluff, more than sixty miles away from their home. The couple managed this long-distance commute until they had their second child, Myra. They wanted to raise their children together, so they moved to Houston, Texas. The booming city allowed Dr. James Jones to work as the associate dean of students at Texas Southern University, only ten minutes' drive from his wife's new residency program. Dr. Irby Jones continued her medical training at Baylor College of Medicine Affiliated Hospitals, where she became the first black woman intern, and only the second black physician, in the internal medicine program, in 1959.[29]

The hospital system maintained policies of racial segregation and limited Dr. Irby Jones to the lesser-resourced integrated hospital. She wasn't allowed to work at the main hospital because it served only white patients. Unwilling to accept subpar medical training, Dr. Irby Jones completed the last three months of her residency at Freedmen's Hospital in Washington, DC, the same hospital that trained Dr. Ferebee and Dr. Edwards.[30] She rejoined her family in Houston once she completed her training.

In 1962, Dr. Irby Jones took the bold step of establishing a private practice in inner city Houston to serve people who didn't have any other access to healthcare, using $17,000 that a local businessman loaned her to open the clinic. At the time, there were only two other black women physicians practicing in Houston: Dr. Thelma Patten Law and Dr. Catherine Roett-Reid.[31] Dr. Irby Jones's clinic helped fulfill her childhood dream of serving people regardless of their ability to pay. She upheld this mission throughout her medical career, expanding her work beyond the US through her involvement in international clinics in Haiti, Mexico, Cuba, China, the Soviet Union, and throughout Africa.

She also advocated for underserved communities through her involvement in organized medicine. In 1985, Dr. Edith Irby Jones became the first woman to serve as president of the National Medical Association, which had been founded in 1895 to support African American physicians who had been excluded from the first medical association in the US—the American Medical Association.[32] (This racial exclusion persisted into the 1960s.)

During her inauguration speech for the National Medical Association, Dr. Irby Jones referenced how her family's own limited access to healthcare had shaped her idea of the role of a physician. "We give little when we give only our material possessions. It is when we give of ourselves that we truly give—the long challenging hours with patients who can pay and those who cannot pay, the agony of sharing the hurts of families with the death of loved ones, the observations of dehumanizing effects of seeing the jobless, the crushed ambitions, and the sharing when all we have to hold on to is the 'being within' to inspire the young to take up our role. We have the comfort of knowing that our work is not to make a living but to make a life, not just for ourselves or a select few, but life with its fullness for all, and especially providing the access to health care, which is our special charge."[33]

Dr. Edith Irby Jones's legacy went beyond her own accomplishments. She became a role model for black girls in the South who had yet to see themselves in medicine. Her presence within the field sparked an interest in some black girls who were headed down a very different career path, providing them the guidance they needed to make their own defining mark on the medical field. One of these black girls grew up to be Dr. Joycelyn Elders, a trailblazer in her own right.

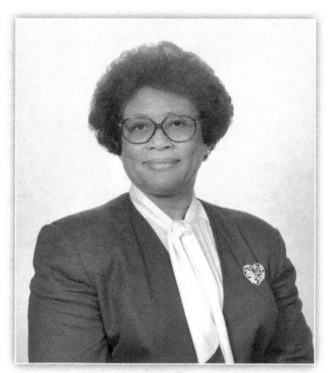

Joycelyn Elders

CHAPTER 6

YOU CAN'T BE WHAT YOU CAN'T SEE

Joycelyn Elders's early childhood was much like Edith Irby Jones's. Born in 1933 in Schaal, Arkansas, six years after Edith, Joycelyn was the daughter of Curtis and Haller Jones, who also worked as sharecroppers. Edith and Joycelyn lived only a three-hour drive from each other. While Edith's father's untimely death abruptly plucked the family from sharecropping and dropped them into an unstable situation, in which they needed to seek support and shelter from extended family, Joycelyn's family stayed firmly entrenched in sharecropping throughout her childhood. The oldest of eight children, Joycelyn juggled the demands of working in the fields while also helping her mom look after her younger siblings.

Even as a child, Joycelyn was up before sunrise to work in the field. Row by row, she would pick the fruit off the plant stem and pull vegetables out of the fertile ground. When the sun beat down on her, she produced more liquid in the sweat pouring down her face than the fruit juice contained in her ripest peaches. And the family was responsible for more than just crops. They also had to raise chickens and hogs, and milk cows to produce precious dairy products. Despite waking up so early, Joycelyn was often still working in the fields once the sun went down, trading the blistering heat for ravenous mosquitos. She started this work when she was just five years old.

At the age when kids become more adept at gross motor skills, like running and jumping, and their brains have developed enough to enable them to count to ten, instead of playing hopscotch and running around on a playground, Joycelyn used her newfound skills to contribute to her struggling family. She would likely have run to the field, plucked the fluffy white cotton from its plant and maybe counted the number of cotton pieces she'd picked, at least up to ten. Any fun that could be gained from gardening was quickly squashed by the immense workload that was necessary to make a dismal income.

Joycelyn's family stretched their earnings as far as they could, but as she would detail in her memoir years later, the family was forced to skip meals on a regular basis. When they ran out of water while enduring the debilitating heat, they suffered from parched mouths and growling stomachs. The family lived without running water or electricity. The sun and candles were their only sources of light. The children quickly learned not to run around the house at night. One innocent misstep could set the entire home aflame. To top it off, their bathrooms were outdoor privies. Fear crept into Joycelyn's consciousness whenever she had to use the privy because screw worms crawling around inside it were as big as baby snakes, threatening to attack if Joycelyn took a wrong step. She kept her trips to the bathroom as efficient as possible to minimize time she spent in close contact with the squirming creatures.[1]

The generational poverty and the demand for young black children to work in the fields, dating back to slavery, hindered Joycelyn's parents from attaining a substantial education. No one in her family had finished high school. Haller, Joycelyn's mother, was able to complete only eighth grade. But Haller wanted Joycelyn to have a better life than hers. She saw education as Joycelyn's way out. Before Joycelyn started school, Haller taught her the alphabet and numbers, and even taught her how to read. She would drill this material into Joycelyn's head, hoping the time spent preparing for school would help Joycelyn overcome the setback of growing up with limited resources.

The training paid off. Joycelyn started school, at five years old, knowing how to read and how to add. Joycelyn internalized the spirit of hard work and determination that her mother taught her. As Joycelyn progressed through school, she remained motivated, despite a suboptimal learning environment. Oftentimes, she had to study in a cramped room that she shared with her sisters. As the night wore on, she would feel chills as the cool night breeze glided in through the broken windows.

Resisting the temptation to curl up under a blanket and fall asleep, Joycelyn would spend hours crouched next to a kerosene lamp studying her school material until she mastered it.[2]

Despite Joycelyn's hard work, the community's limited resources affected the quality of its education system, making it harder for children in Joycelyn's small town to advance. Her first school was a one-room schoolhouse. The four walls threatened to suffocate the intellectual potential of its students as one teacher, Miss Brown, strove to teach students ranging from five to eighteen years of age within one space. With each age group at drastically different stages of development, chaos was inevitable. The younger kids would get bored with their assignments within a few minutes, preferring to run and play around in the classroom, just as the teenagers were beginning to focus on their own work.

There were only about twenty students in the classroom. Still, Miss Brown struggled to manage the strikingly different intellectual and developmental stages of her students. She needed to employ the help of some of her more advanced students, even though this could slow the progress that those students made in school. Joycelyn became one of her little helpers; she was even assigned to help kids who were older than she was. When the older students should've been reading complex sentence structures, Joycelyn was responsible for teaching them the basics. Limited educational support, coupled with the demands of field work, stunted the intellectual development of many of these children. Joycelyn was so busy trying to help the kids who were behind, it was difficult for her to stay on track, much less advance.

Things weren't as hectic for every primary school in the 1930s. It was something that many poor black communities dealt with, while the white communities benefited from more educational support. As was commonplace for many of the schools in the Jim Crow South, Joycelyn's primary school received resources, such as books, after the schools for white children were done with them, and many books were received ragged and worn. Hand-me-downs were the school's only option, and the books were reused year after year. The kids cherished them because they were all that they had.

Fighting an uphill battle, Joycelyn not only had to navigate limited resources at her school; she also had to manage the competing priorities of being a child in a farming family. Many of the kids at Joycelyn's school had this heavy burden on their shoulders. In the early spring, when it was time to plant the crops, school was put on hold. Joycelyn and the other children in farming families could only go back to school once the field work was done. She would catch up on what she had missed. And then—boom!—she was out of school again in the fall to gather the crops. Every year, this debilitating cycle. Her ability to go to school and make progress with her education was dictated by the seasons and the demands of the crops in her family's field. This pattern continued through high school. Joycelyn was so proud when she reached milestones in the field, like being able to pick two hundred pounds of cotton a day. This increased efficiency in the field brought her one step closer to breaking through the wall that had kept her family and many of her community members at or below eighth-grade education levels.

While learning grammar and arithmetic, Joycelyn also learned the consequences of being a poor black person in America. Her family had learned how to live without electricity, running water, and indoor plumbing. They went without these things for most of Joycelyn's childhood and adolescence. But there was one thing that was almost impossible to live without: healthcare. Without access to medical care, Joycelyn's family survived off of home remedies. Castor oil, turpentine, and quinine. Even kerosene on sugar cubes. Whenever a family member fell ill, the house would fill with the distinct smells of medicinal concoctions whose recipes had been passed down from generation to generation.

These practices were essential to the African American community in the antebellum period, when white people didn't allow African Americans to receive regular medical care. During this time, the African Americans who had the greatest exposure to doctors were those who were forced or tricked into becoming subjects of experiments that carried great risk and that were conducted with the goal of developing safer treatments for white patients. Even after the Emancipation Proclamation was signed, African American families were severely restricted from accessing healthcare because of policies of racial segregation at hospitals and by the complete refusal of some hospitals even to treat African American patients. Again, the African American patients who received the most medical attention were the ones who were treated as guinea pigs for experimental treatments, oftentimes without their knowledge or consent. In these conditions, many African American families were forced to rely on do-it-yourself healthcare, including ingredients and practices that would be hazardous if used incorrectly.

In a 2008 interview, Joycelyn well remembered the one time her family diverged from this mode of medical care: when her baby brother became gravely ill. His abdomen was distended, looking like a grown man's beer belly would after the man had downed a case of Budweiser. He was experiencing a dull pain, which grew worse in tandem with his waistline. He felt nauseous and didn't want to eat, and his forehead was burning hot to the touch. But the most concerning sign of all was that he was the only one in the family who was sick. With the common cold or food poisoning, the whole family would have become ill. This time, it was just the brother. Joycelyn remembered her mom, Haller, being filled with worry. Breaking from their norm, Haller told her husband, "Curtis, you're gonna have to take my baby to the doctor."[3]

Hastily, Curtis constructed a makeshift saddle and placed it on his mule for his son to sit on. Together, they took a miserable thirteen-mile mule ride to the nearest doctor. Each gallop the mule took sent a sharp pain through the boy's body. Curtis and his son finally made it to the doctor's office, but they weren't seen immediately. There were white patients there, and they were the doctor's top priority. It didn't matter that some of the white patients had arrived at the doctor's office hours after Curtis and his son. The white patients were to be seen first. Once all of the white patients had been seen, if the office was still open, the doctor would begin seeing the black patients.

So after that difficult journey to see the doctor, they waited all day to receive medical care. When the doctor got to Joycelyn's brother, the sun was beginning to set. Upon examination of the boy, the doctor realized that the child likely had a dangerous infection in the lower right quadrant of his abdomen, but the doctor didn't have much time to address the issue. He hurriedly sliced open the boy's abdomen and inserted a drainage tube. Yellow-tinged creamy pus quickly drained out. This invasive procedure came with some serious health risks. If Joycelyn's brother had been white, he would've been admitted into the hospital to be watched by a medical team to ensure that nothing went wrong. But the affiliated hospitals refused to treat black patients, so this sick child was sent back home. Still feeling weak and nauseous, the boy rode back home with his dad. A rubber tube protruded from his abdomen, and each galloping step from the mule sent another surge of pain through his body, and more pus spluttered out.[4]

The family's prayers were answered when their baby boy slowly recovered. Looking back on this experience, Dr. Elders believed that her younger brother had had appendicitis. She believed his appendix had ruptured and caused peritonitis, an infection in his peritoneum, which is a serous membrane that lines the abdominal cavity. This kind of infection can be fatal.

In the case of a life-threatening condition like this, Joycelyn's brother should have received much better care. But the family experienced conditions that many black families were forced to live through, especially when the only doctors they had access to were white men who upheld racist discriminatory practices. With such limited access to medical care, this was the only medical encounter Joycelyn was exposed to while she was growing up. In her opinion, her brother was "treated like a pig."[5] While this likely brought her pain and resentment, she didn't have time to sulk over the cruel treatment that poor black families like hers had to endure. She needed to stay focused on her studies. This was the key to a better life for herself and her family.

Joycelyn was driven by having seven younger siblings who looked up to her and two parents who encouraged her pursuit of a more extensive education. With this motivation, she far outpaced her family's educational level when she graduated from high school at age fourteen. And she didn't just get through high school; Joycelyn excelled. She maintained a strong academic record despite her responsibilities at home, caring for her younger siblings, and at the plantation, and graduated as her high school's valedictorian.[6]

Joycelyn and her family were elated. This was a huge milestone, and it set an example for her younger siblings. On her graduation day, Joycelyn was approached by a representative of Philander Smith College, a historically black college in Little Rock, Arkansas. The man revealed that since Joycelyn was the highest-ranked student in her class, she was eligible for a scholarship from the United Methodist Women that offered full tuition to Philander Smith College. The generosity changed her life. Reflecting back on that moment, Joycelyn recalled, "Well, I was thrilled to death, but I didn't know—I didn't know what that meant. And what I mean by that—I didn't know you had to apply to college. I didn't know, you know, you had to get to college. I didn't know anything."[7] Coming from a family who didn't have experience with higher education, and from a high school that was under-resourced (as most black schools in the Jim Crow South were), Joycelyn didn't have the support she needed to seamlessly transition to college. Despite the tuition scholarship, Joycelyn still had financial and institutional hurdles that she had to overcome.

Because her hometown was a small community with fewer than a hundred residents, everyone heard that Joycelyn was going to college, so, just as Edith Irby's community had for her, they did their best to help Joycelyn prepare. Her neighbors were also poor and couldn't afford nice clothes for themselves, but they wanted Joycelyn to have these niceties when she went to school. Some families pooled their money to buy Joycelyn a handkerchief. She also received a pair of shoes with black and white trimming. Her family even spent part of the summer picking peaches to buy plaid fabric, which her aunt used to make her a colorful dress. This was all she had. Her aunts from Detroit added to this collection by sending her cast-off clothes from the families they worked for.

The recycled clothes were some of the nicest Joycelyn ever owned. As she packed her new fancy clothes into an old, dilapidated suitcase that she borrowed from her grandmother, she was filled with excitement. But she still needed to find a way to actually get to the school, which was about 150 miles from home. There was a bus that went to Little Rock, but it would cost her $3.43. A poor sharecropping family, the Elderses did not have that much in disposable income to pay for her trip, but they were determined to get Joycelyn to Little Rock. The entire family, including her younger siblings, worked overtime in the fields to raise enough money for her bus ticket. Joycelyn remembered it vividly. After spending all day picking cotton, her five-year-old brother looked up to her and asked, "Do we have enough yet?"[8]

His words stung her heart. She didn't want her younger siblings working like dogs so that she could go to school. In response, she made a promise to herself. "I didn't say anything to anybody, but I said, 'I'll make sure that all of my sisters and brothers that want to go to college or want to get away, I'll find a way to help them.' And you know, I'm rather proud of me: I did."[9]

The members of this family were committed to supporting one another. While Joycelyn's parents didn't have the experience that would allow them to advise her on the process of getting to college, or on how to be successful there, they did what they could to help her achieve her goals. Once Joycelyn shattered the academic barrier, she served as an example for the rest of her siblings. She showed them it was possible. Because many of her siblings followed in her footsteps and went to college, this lone United Methodist Women's scholarship essentially helped the entire family transcend extreme poverty. A single initiative that sought to support children from underserved communities helped to undo some of the harm caused by the systemic oppression that plagued this family since their ancestors were forced into slavery.

The young Joycelyn took the long bus ride by herself and arrived at Philander Smith College thrilled to start a new chapter in her life. Bags in hand, she hiked up to the admissions office to find out about her living accommodations and class schedule. The college administrators searched for her file but couldn't find her name. Even after checking a number of locations in the office, in case her file had been misplaced, they came up empty. The admissions office reached out to administrators in other departments, but no one knew who Joycelyn was. With each failed attempt to find her file, Joycelyn felt her excitement undermined by panic. Why couldn't they find her information?

When the admissions officers asked Joycelyn a few questions, they reached the root of the problem: Joycelyn hadn't submitted an application to Philander Smith College. But no one told her that she had needed to! They had only offered her the scholarship and told her when to arrive at the school. The man at her high school graduation probably assumed that she understood the college application process. But Joycelyn didn't know that she needed to apply to college. She hadn't had to apply to high school. Why would she need to apply to college? Joycelyn didn't have a college advisor at her high school, or insider knowledge from her family. Afraid that this simple mistake had just cost her the only shot she had at a college education, Joycelyn was filled with sorrow. In this new town, all alone and without the money to take the bus back home, this fourteen-year-old child went to a windowsill in the middle of the college hall and began sobbing.[10] It seemed as though her bright future had just crumbled before her eyes.

Her solitary grieving was interrupted when the president of the college, Dr. Marquis Lafayette Harris, walked by. He was concerned, and he asked her why she was so sad. Joycelyn explained her dire situation. The sky was growing dark, and options were dwindling by the minute. Conscious of the time crunch, the president instructed Joycelyn to go to the girls dormitory while he took care of the matter. Within the day, he sorted the paperwork with the admissions office so that Joycelyn could attend Philander Smith College.

This kind of goodwill is a defining feature of historically black colleges and universities. They have sought to support children who come from difficult situations like Joycelyn's. Although such students don't always have the resources to produce gleaming résumés and college essays, or even know how to apply to college in the first place, HBCUs have seen their potential and helped them overcome their situations. Joycelyn's situation was not the most extreme example of this altruism because she had a scholarship from a foundation that was affiliated with the university. Still, this general philosophy of supporting black students, even if they aren't polished when they start at a school, is upheld by HBCUs. The practice has helped many iconic leaders, such as Oprah

Winfrey and Toni Morrison, reach their potential, even though their upbringings made it more difficult for them to have successful careers.

When Joycelyn received the opportunity to attend college, her plan was to earn her bachelor's degree and then secure a job as a salesclerk at a Dillard's store in Nashville. This was her dream. She explained: "If I got a job working as a clerk in [a] Dillard's store, I would've died and gone to heaven. [Then], at least I would get out of the hot sun."[11] Although working as a salesclerk wasn't the highest-earning job, it offered the financial independence that sharecropping didn't. As sharecroppers, her family was always indebted to the landowner. He could kick them off his land without warning or raise the cost to rent the land without increasing compensation for the crops that they were harvesting. Salesclerks earned significantly more money than sharecroppers did, and their quality of life was better.

As Joycelyn progressed through college, she began to consider a different route. After taking a chemistry class that she found interesting, she played with the idea of becoming a laboratory technician. Even though Joycelyn excelled in her classes, a high-ranked position in the sciences seemed out of reach, because she hadn't been exposed to anyone like her who had been that successful. This all changed after she joined Delta Sigma Theta Sorority in the spring semester of her freshman year.

Delta Sigma Theta, the black sorority that Edith Irby Jones had joined early in her college career, was founded in 1913, five years after Alpha Kappa Alpha was established. Like Dr. Dorothy Ferebee, who had participated in community service work as a member of Alpha Kappa Alpha, Joycelyn served her community through her sorority. Delta Sigma Theta brought black women leaders to campus to speak to the student body. During her sophomore year, Joycelyn organized an event at which Edith, a medical student at the time, came to speak. Joycelyn was completely captivated when this black woman medical student, only a few years older, encouraged Joycelyn and the other attendees to strive to be the best that they could be. Joycelyn recalled the pivotal moment: "From that moment on, all I could dream about was I wanted to be just like her. . . . You see, I had never seen a doctor before I went to college; and you can't be what you can't see."[12]

Both Edith and Joycelyn had challenging upbringings that made it unlikely that they would overcome poverty, let alone become physicians. Even though the young women were extremely intelligent and hardworking, the socioeconomic status of their families, combined with their race and gender, erected many barriers that made social mobility nearly impossible. Immense family and community support helped them to continue their success in school, and unlikely experiences fixed them on the path toward medicine. For Edith, that experience was the loss of her sister to typhoid fever, when the doctor didn't provide as much medical care as he could have because Edith's family was poor. For Joycelyn, it was meeting Edith. This was the first time she saw what a physician looked like, and, incredibly, that physician looked like her. The simple meeting redefined in Joycelyn's mind the possibilities for her future.

Once Joycelyn decided that she wanted to become a physician, she had to figure out how she would pay for medical school. She couldn't rely on her parents. They were still struggling to take care of her seven younger siblings. After thinking through her limited options, Joycelyn came up with a solution. She would join the army. Thanks to the GI Bill, Joycelyn's service bought financial support for medical school. She joined the Women's Army Specialist Corps, which allowed her to train as a physical therapist at the Brooke Army Medical Center at Fort Sam Houston, Texas.

It was yet another opportunity for Joycelyn to expand her horizons. The student population at her college was composed primarily of African Americans from low-income backgrounds, but her military unit was filled with white women from middle- and upper-income families. She learned how to work with them, and she gained insight from their perspectives on life. During her military service, she also had the chance to explore new cities around the country, opportunities that took her far outside her comfort zone and into exciting new territory. The experience confirmed her desire to establish a career beyond the confines of her small community. Joycelyn explained: "I was like a sponge. I absorbed everything around me, and I knew one thing absolute. I never wanted to go back to the farm."[13]

In 1956, after she had served in the army for three years, Joycelyn went back to Arkansas to start medical school at the University of Arkansas College of Medicine. It was just four years after Dr. Edith Irby Jones had graduated from the school. In Joycelyn's class, there were about a hundred medical students, including three black students and three female students. Joycelyn, as the only black woman in her class, was at the intersection of these two identities. While the University of Arkansas medical school had trained other black students since Dr. Irby Jones broke the color line, the students had all been black men. Joycelyn was the second black woman to train at the school.[14]

Joycelyn's medical school experience shared many similarities with Dr. Irby Jones's. When she encountered racism or sexism at medical school, she employed strategies similar to the ones Dr. Irby Jones had used by reframing the prejudiced behavior so that it wouldn't weigh her down or threaten her goal of becoming a physician. Her experience growing up in the South had desensitized her to many forms of racism. She described a poignant experience that many would have found offensive but which she instead chose to brush off: "I remember my next door [neighbor]—a lady, a white lady who lived across the street from us. She would help my mom. She was wonderful. But . . . she was always talking about—even after I was Surgeon General—that I was her little n*gger girl. Well, I could've been offended by that, but she'd done that all of her life. . . . She really meant it being proud of me. At least that—I don't know how she meant it. That's how I accepted it, that she was really very proud of me. I was always so grateful how much she, you know, with eight babies and all that—how much she had helped my mother, you know, when she would have her babies. . . . So, the fact that she called me her little n*gger girl never, never bothered me, because I thought about the good things that she'd done for my mother in the past."[15]

Joycelyn grew up around people who made boldly racist comments toward her, even as they claimed to care about her. But this contradictory behavior was not unusual. People like Joycelyn's white neighbor were products of a larger social structure that was deeply embedded with racist and sexist attitudes. These attitudes influenced the rules at her medical school. As with Edith, the three black students in Joycelyn's medical class were not allowed to eat in the dining room that was desig-nated for medical students because the white students ate there. Joycelyn and the other two black students had to eat where the janitors and cooks ate. But when she reflected on her time in medical school, Joycelyn didn't categorize this as racism. It was just life. When someone grows up in a hate-filled environment, where racism is literally codified in law, how can they distinguish between "normal" acceptable behavior and problematic behavior that they might want to speak out against?

Even when Joycelyn did identify someone as racist, she had to de-cide how she would respond. She would have been completely justified in feeling hurt and upset by these experiences. But when someone is constantly bombarded with racist encounters, the pain of responding to those situations can be exhausting. By the time Joycelyn made it to medical school, she had to figure out how to navigate being a black woman and being a medical student. Medical school can be emotion-ally draining all by itself. If a black woman medical student lets every hateful comment affect her, she might not make it through her training. Joycelyn was not willing to let other people's prejudice prevent her from accomplishing her goal. She kept her blinders on, deflecting any negativ-ity, as she continued to plow forward toward her destiny.

In her final years of medical school, Joycelyn met her future hus-band, Oliver Elders. He was the basketball coach at Horace Mann High School, the only black high school in Little Rock, and Joycelyn was as-signed to perform medical examinations on the players.[16] When Joyce-lyn first showed up at basketball practice, Oliver thought she was lost and needed to be directed to a different part of the school. When Joyce-lyn explained that she was the doctor sent to examine his players, Oliver was shocked. Forty years later, he recalled how he felt in that moment: "Well, my mouth was open, and I couldn't close it, because up till then I had literally never heard of a lady doctor. I thought that doctors were males."[17]

This misconception about who could be a doctor was likely pervasive in many parts of the US, even in the second half of the twentieth century. Some people would resist the idea that women doctors existed, but Oli-ver quickly accepted this reality, and his surprise suddenly transformed into intrigue. He gave Joycelyn a season pass to the team's games as a thank-you for completing their medical exams, then he asked her on a date. Their romance quickly blossomed. One day, Oliver was driving Joycelyn to Minnesota for a residency interview; two months later, they were married. Four months after that, in June 1960, Dr. Joycelyn Elders graduated from the University of Arkansas School of Medicine.

Once Joycelyn was married, she began the juggling act that most women struggle with when they want both a family and a career. She initially sought a spot at the University of Minnesota, which was known to have a great pediatric residency program, and she wanted to become a pediatric surgeon. Numerous mentors had encouraged her to continue her clinical training there, confident that it would boost her career. As she went through the residency application process, she grew increasingly excited about the prospect of moving to Minnesota. So when she received her acceptance from Minnesota's pediatric program, she should've been elated. Instead, she worried about how her career advancement could negatively impact her marriage.

Oliver planned to keep his coaching job in Arkansas, so if Joycelyn accepted the internship spot in Minnesota, they would have to spend at least a year separated by almost nine hundred miles. It was an extremely hard decision for Joycelyn because she and Oliver didn't want to be separated from each other, especially when they were still newlyweds. She ended up accepting the internship because they both agreed it would be best for the family. But she admitted thinking, "If I had known I was going to fall in love with someone whose career was in Arkansas, I most likely never would have even thought about Minnesota."[18]

Traditionally, when both partners in a heteronormative relationship have careers, the burden usually falls on the woman to make professional sacrifices to protect the relationship, while the man is allowed to do what's best for his career. The argument that some men make is that they are the primary breadwinners in their homes, so a good job move for them is also good for their families. Because Dr. Elders was the primary breadwinner in her household, she felt comfortable accepting the internship position in Minnesota based on this logic. But she didn't keep this mentality for long.

Dr. Elders was a great intern in Minnesota, so much so that the school offered her a spot in its competitive residency program. This would allow her to pursue her dream of becoming a pediatric surgeon, but it would mean spending five to six years in Minnesota. Dr. Elders believed that her husband would've moved to Minnesota if she had pushed the issue, but she didn't push it. Oliver was on track to becoming a great basketball coach in Arkansas, and she didn't want to take that from him. While he could've had a successful coaching career in Minnesota too, Dr. Elders thought asking him to move "wouldn't have just been senseless and unfair; it would have been cruel."[19] So she put the advancement of her husband's career over her own. She turned down the offer at the University of Minnesota and let go of her aspirations of becoming a pediatric surgeon. Instead, she completed a pediatric residency at the University of Arkansas. Because the school didn't have a pediatric surgery program, she instead trained to become a pediatric endocrinologist.

While Joycelyn showed her support for her husband's career by making this sacrifice, Oliver displayed his devotion to Joycelyn and her career pursuits by being her rock during the more treacherous seasons of her career journey, such as during her postgraduate clinical training. The pediatric program at the University of Arkansas required its residents to work insane hours, a practice that is slowly changing. Dr. Elders would regularly have to work thirty-six hours straight at the hospital, staying at the hospital every third night. And when she was allowed to go home, she was usually on call. This meant that if an emergency came up while she was home, she was expected to go back to the hospital and stay there until the matter was resolved, even though those nights were meant to be her rest nights.[20] Dr. Elders faced intense stress and sleep deprivation as she went through the process, so Oliver supported her by going to the hospital every time she was set to spend the night there. Whether it was a twenty-minute conversation or a quick meal, the quality time with her husband helped Dr. Elders decompress and regain her energy so that she could provide quality care for her next patients.

Oliver's support was Dr. Elders's lifeline when she struggled to cope with some of the more difficult cases. That of a thirteen-year-old girl, whom she called Mary (which may be an alias to preserve the patient's privacy), is one that she would never forget. Mary presented with bulging eyes and a large goiter on her neck, which is indicative of thyroid enlargement. This clinical presentation made the medical team think that she might be suffering from hyperthyroidism. In addition to these symptoms, Mary suffered from high blood pressure, severe nervousness, bed-wetting, weight loss, and poor school performance. After the team of physicians confirmed that Mary had hyperthyroidism, they kept her in the hospital for two weeks to treat her illness.

Dr. Elders and Mary developed a friendship during her stay. When the team thought Mary was stable enough to be discharged, Dr. Elders excitedly went to go tell her the news. From experience, Dr. Elders knew that most children were elated to go home. But this wasn't the case with Mary. She started sobbing and confessed that she didn't want to go home. Dr. Elders became concerned and asked Mary why she felt this way. While Mary was hesitant to tell Dr. Elders what was wrong, she eventually confided in her: "Saturday nights my Daddy and my brother and my uncles use me. . . . They use me and my sister. Saturdays is when they get drunk. They take me and my sister out back and they get on us."[21]

Distraught over this heart-wrenching revelation, Dr. Elders rushed to the hospital's social worker for advice. She wanted to report this sexual abuse to the police, but she was advised against it. (This was about five years before Arkansas changed its laws to require doctors to report suspected child abuse. Until the legislation, most doctors didn't report suspected abuse. If they did, the families could sue them, and the doctors could face legal repercussions.) All Dr. Elders could do was talk to a family member deemed safe to speak with and see if the person would take action. Dr. Elders brought up her concerns to Mary's mother, but the mother brushed off what was happening to her daughters, claiming, "Some of them liked to go out and drink a little home brew on Saturdays and have a little fun. But they weren't doing anything where someone could get hurt."[22] To Dr. Elders, this response corroborated Mary's account, but indicated that the mother didn't want to do anything to help her daughters. So Dr. Elders was forced to send Mary back into that abusive home environment.

Dr. Elders was able to see Mary only two more times for follow-up visits. During her last visit, she found out that Mary was pregnant by one of the men who raped her. In that part of the country in the 1960s, if a teenage girl got pregnant and wasn't married, her "life was considered ruined."[23] It didn't matter that Mary was a victim and that what had happened occurred without her consent—she would be blamed and punished by society. And she would have to have the baby because abortion was not an option. At that time, abortion was illegal in Arkansas, regardless of the reason. It didn't matter that this child was raped or that the conception came about through incest. The thirteen-year-old girl would have to figure out a way to support herself and the child. Over her multiple decades in pediatrics, Dr. Elders saw many children in horrifying situations like this one. These experiences shaped her views on how medical and educational institutions should care for children, driving her farther away from the conservative views that were more prevalent in the South.

Once Joycelyn adjusted to the demands of her residency program, she and Oliver began to grow their family. They had their first child, Eric, when Joycelyn was in her second year of residency. She continued seeing patients throughout her pregnancy, even on a day when she was in active labor, but she happily took her six weeks of maternity leave once her son was born. After completing her residency, Dr. Elders started a three-year research fellowship and junior faculty position. During this time, she had her second child, Kevin. Dr. Elders found it challenging caring for two babies during the early stages of her career, but as her sons grew older and she became more settled in her academic positions, things got easier. She settled into her work routine and remained determined to help children and educate a new generation of doctors.

In 1986, after more than twenty-five years as a physician, Dr. Elders received a surprise call from the governor of Arkansas, Bill Clinton. He asked if she would consider being the director of the Arkansas Department of Health. She was hesitant to agree because she was very happy with her job. She was a practicing pediatric endocrinologist who also conducted clinical research in pediatrics and taught medical students at the University of Arkansas. It was the career she had dreamed about since she had first met Dr. Edith Irby Jones. She didn't want to leave her job. Because she respected Governor Clinton, she told him she would consider his offer if he met several conditions, including the ability to retain her position at the medical center and a 10 percent raise.

She thought these requirements would be too difficult for him to meet, so she forgot about his offer and was content to continue working in her position at the University of Arkansas. Two or three weeks later, Governor Clinton called her in the middle of the night to tell her that he would agree to her terms. He asked if she would accept his offer. Flustered and still half asleep, she began her response saying that she liked to keep her word. He took that as an acceptance of the position and hung up the phone before she could come up with a reason why she couldn't take the position. After talking it over with her mother and some trusted colleagues, Dr. Elders became convinced that she could continue to make an impact in areas that she cared about, such as adolescent health and teenage pregnancy, if she led the state health department.

When she began her work as director, Arkansas had the second-highest rate of teenage pregnancy in the country, high rates of AIDS, low levels of education, and high levels of poverty.[24] During her first year at the department, she visited different counties in the state to better understand the problems. When she visited Governor Clinton's hometown, Hope, where she spoke to a group of high school boys, she was shocked by their misconceptions around safe sex and family planning. They thought that they couldn't get a girl pregnant if they had sex while standing up. They also thought that condoms would tighten around their penis and, if they used condoms too much, their penises would rot off.[25] Due to these pervasive myths, many kids were having unprotected sex, making them susceptible to unwanted pregnancies and sexually transmitted infections. Meeting the locals there, as well as in many other counties, convinced her that she needed to make strong efforts to address these issues.

Dr. Elders tells a story of a time, only three weeks into her job as director, when her unique methods of effecting change caused a stir. She was meeting with Clinton and several other leaders of the governor's administration to discuss youth and families. When Dr. Elders was asked what the health department was going to do to help this population, she said that they were going to work to prevent teenage pregnancies.

Immediately, the media pounced: "Well, Dr. Elders, how do you plan to do that?"

She came up with a quick response. "We're gonna have a health education . . . in schools and teach, you know, comprehensive health education in schools and . . . school-based clinics."

Struck by the idea of comprehensive health education for kids, the reporter prompted, "Are you going to have condoms at school?"

Confident in her stance, Dr. Elders replied, "Well, we aren't going to put them on their lunch plate, but yes."[26]

This response caused a sudden flurry among the reporters. As they turned to see how Clinton reacted, his face turned beet red. While Clinton's response wasn't as blunt as hers, Dr. Elders felt that it still conveyed support for what she was saying. It was all the approval she needed to keep working to address the problems in Arkansas, despite what the media had to say about her. Throughout her six-year tenure, she and the rest of the department worked tirelessly to help their community. By the time Dr. Elders finished her tenure, she had helped reduce the teen-pregnancy rate through sex education in schools and the increased availability of birth control. She established programs to reduce both violence against women and child abuse. She raised the state's childhood immunization rate from 34 percent to 60 percent. And she made various other improvements in the health conditions of Arkansas residents.[27]

Shortly after Clinton was elected president of the United States, in 1992, he invited Dr. Elders to the governor's mansion. There, he asked if she would be his surgeon general, so that she could have the same impact in Washington that she had had in Arkansas. Again, she was reluctant. She loved her job as director of the Arkansas Department of Health. But after spending some time reflecting on the president-elect's offer, she happily accepted the position. She became the first African American, and the second woman, to be appointed surgeon general of the United States of America.

Working as director of the Arkansas Department of Health had pushed Dr. Elders outside of her comfort zone, and so did her work as surgeon general, but she quickly grew to love it. The position allowed her to have a positive impact on the whole nation. She sought to address such issues as teenage pregnancy and access to healthcare, and the HIV/AIDS epidemic. She wanted to help the entire nation, but she also recognized that such issues disproportionately affected the African American community. At the state health department, she led various health initiatives, but her position as surgeon general was more about using her platform to share the White House's stance on various health issues, with the goal of influencing policy in the administration's favor. Throughout her time in the role, Dr. Elders gave on average twenty speeches per month around the country.[28]

Having so much exposure gave Dr. Elders ample opportunity to comment on controversial topics, which could land her in newspaper headlines. She was a passionate physician at heart, not a politician. She didn't worry about determining the most diplomatic way to discuss issues like sex education and HIV/AIDS prevention; she just said what she thought and felt. Sometimes she said brash things, like, "We've taught teenagers what to do in the front seat of cars, now we have to teach them what to do in the back."[29] She meant, of course, that we've spent a lot of time teaching teenagers how to drive safely, but it's just as important that we teach them about safe sex, to prevent unwanted pregnancies or sexually transmitted infections like HIV/AIDS. Her language was memorable, if not delicate.

Sometimes her comments were taken out of context. For instance, she spoke at a United Nations conference that was focused on the AIDS epidemic and the need to fight the taboo of talking about sex. During one session, a psychiatrist spoke about the prospect of masturbation as a safer form of sexual release that could possibly reduce the rate of HIV/AIDS. When he asked Dr. Elders if there should be more discussion around and promotion of masturbation, she said that masturbation "is part of human sexuality, and it's a part of something that perhaps should be taught. But we've not even taught our children the very basics.

And I feel that we have tried ignorance for a very long time and it's time we try education."[30] Following this conversation, she was accused of encouraging the teaching of masturbation in schools. Eventually, controversy around Dr. Elders's liberal views built up so much that she was considered a liability to the Clinton administration. On December 9, 1994, Dr. Elders was asked to resign, after fifteen months as surgeon general.

While she was disappointed that her time in Washington ended the way it had, she didn't regret standing up for what she believed. So many people in the country were struggling because they weren't receiving proper medical education or resources, and Dr. Elders saw it as her job to stand boldly for those people, rather than worry about how to navigate the maze of political niceties. After she resigned, she returned to her job as a pediatric endocrinologist at the University of Arkansas and continued her advocacy work. Even today, in her late eighties, she still gives talks around the country, inspiring many.

Dr. Joycelyn Elders's journey in medicine began with an encounter with a successful black woman in medicine. Seeing Dr. Edith Irby Jones was like being shown a magical mirror; she saw that it was possible for someone like her to achieve great things, to contribute to her community and even her country. Now, Dr. Joycelyn Elders serves as that mirror holder for young black women like me.

Only a month into my first year of medical school, I had the honor of virtually streaming into a panel discussion about health disparities that have been made glaringly obvious with the COVID-19 pandemic. All the panelists were former surgeons general. There, Dr. Joycelyn Elders sat among other trailblazing surgeons general, such as Dr. David Satcher and Dr. Antonia Novello. Seeing Dr. Elders in that position suddenly expanded the future I could envision for myself.

Will I become a surgeon general or hold another position that allows me to make a significant impact on my national and even global community? Maybe so. My ambitions don't have to be curtailed because

I'm African American and a woman. I will dream big and hope that the social and structural barriers that make it hard for people like me to succeed will not prevent me from reaching my potential. When Dr. Elders reflected on how much meeting Dr. Irby Jones impacted her career path, she declared, "You can't be what you can't see."[31] Thankfully, I have role models like them to show me that so much is possible for a black woman in medicine.

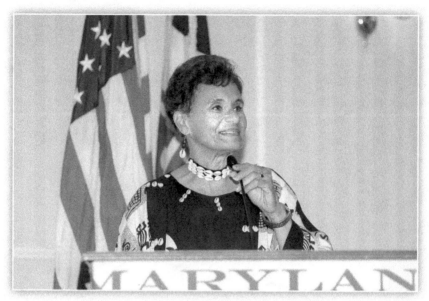

Dr. Marilyn Hughes Gaston

HEALTHCARE IS A HUMAN RIGHT

Marilyn Hughes Gaston was born in 1939, six years after Joycelyn Elders, in Cincinnati, Ohio. Like many other African American women in this lineage, Marilyn came from humble beginnings. The family lived cramped together in an apartment in the projects, with three dilapidated rooms.[1] This was where Dorothy Hughes, Marilyn's mother, went into labor without another soul in sight. Neither the doctor nor her husband and the rest of her family were able to get to her in time, so Dorothy went through the process alone and somehow delivered a healthy baby without any complications. This was how Marilyn entered the world, without access to medical care.

The family continued to struggle with finances, and thus a lack of healthcare, throughout Marilyn's childhood. Unable to afford insurance, they had a minuscule fund for doctors' visits. Dorothy prioritized the care of her children and her husband, Myron Hughes, over her own. Eventually, this caught up with her. On an arid day, when the family was together in their living room, Dorothy just fainted. Marilyn's shock from seeing her mother fall lifelessly to the ground seared this episode into her memory. Forced to finally take Dorothy in to see a doctor, the family learned that she suffered from anemia, a low red blood cell count, due to a worsening cervical cancer. Her brain hadn't received enough oxygen due to the low red blood cell and hemoglobin counts, causing her to faint.

While Marilyn was only a child, she understood that her mom, Dorothy, had become extremely sick because she couldn't afford to see a doctor. It was at this point, when Marilyn was almost ten years old, that she decided to become a doctor. But not just any doctor. Like Dr. Ferebee, Dr. Edwards, and Dr. Irby Jones, Marilyn would dedicate her career to serving poor, uninsured, underserved people. She wanted to do anything she could to prevent what happened to her mom from happening to someone else.

By the time Marilyn reached high school, she was already exhibiting her impressive intellectual capabilities. Although the family was still poor, Marilyn was able to gain access to a prestigious college prep school through her strong performance on its admission test. Given the resources at this school, Marilyn figured that if she told her counselors about her medical aspirations, they would help her reach her goal. Instead, they tried to dissuade her from pursuing a career in medicine. In a 2011 interview, Marilyn still remembered their disparaging words: "Well, you're a Negro . . . and Negros don't get into medical school. . . . Second, you're a woman, and there are very few women in medicine at this time. Third, you are poor. You can't afford it."[2] While it is true that wealthy white men did predominate in medicine during this time, comments like this served only to worsen this demographic discrepancy. While activism and legislation in the 1950s was moving toward a more inclusive education system, Marilyn's experience shows that a black girl could attend a well-resourced racially integrated school and still receive less educational support due to her identities.

If these counselors had been Marilyn's only support, she likely would've abandoned her lofty career aspirations. Thankfully, like Drs. Ferebee, Irby Jones, and Elders before her, she wasn't alone. Marilyn's immediate and extended family supported her goals. Even though they came from difficult circumstances, they were fighters. As Marilyn put it, she was raised by "some fierce black women" and a father who wanted the best for his children.[3] Her parents were activists in their community before the civil rights movement. Marilyn even remembers her godmother becoming president of a local chapter of the NAACP.[4] Marilyn's family's advocacy work against injustice within the community planted the seed of resilience within her. They taught her that she had to believe her dreams were possible regardless of what other people said. This was her compass. It helped her to remain confident in her abilities, even as she navigated a sea of detractors and academic advisors who didn't offer adequate support.

Marilyn stayed local for the early stages of her training. She studied zoology at Miami University in Ohio before studying medicine at the University of Cincinnati College of Medicine, graduating in 1960 and 1964, respectively. When Marilyn started medical school, she was immediately confronted with the realities of systemic oppression. The makeup of her medical class, upon entering in 1960, mirrored that of May Chinn's 1922 medical class on entering medical school: there were only five other women in the class of about a hundred students, and only three African Americans out of the four hundred students who made up the student body.[5]

These skewed demographics had a profound impact on her experiences in medical school. Imagine being in Marilyn's shoes. You decide to pursue a highly regarded career path. After long hours of studying and countless tests, you make it to the final stage of training necessary to make your dream come true. To your surprise, none of the other trainees or professionals look like you. As you try to learn their ways, naturally you feel like an outsider. You might even question why you're there. Do you hold a legitimate place in this community? Even if your skills are on par with those of your fellow trainees, your identities draw you apart. This feeling of not belonging, despite earning one's spot, is the experience of many underrepresented minorities within medicine. It's often labeled "imposter syndrome." It's a debilitating feeling that Marilyn likely wrestled with as well.

But she didn't have the luxury of focusing on any doubts in her mind. She had to worry about the taunts from her colleagues. Many of her white male classmates felt compelled to tease the few female medical students on a regular basis. The men teased the women while the women practiced their clinical skills, and they questioned the women's credibility during discussions of cases. Those were the typical kinds of jokes that the white women experienced. But the men chose a more sinister tone for Marilyn. To them, she wasn't just intellectually incapable of being their medical colleague; she was their sexual plaything. Even when Marilyn was in her seventies, the episodes of sexual harassment reverberated loudly in her mind. "They always teased me in a sexual way. . . . They would ask me questions like 'What do virgins eat for breakfast?' And if you said, 'I don't know,' then you were saying you weren't a virgin and then they would say, 'Well, let's get together.'"[6] While Marilyn might've felt compelled to report the sexual harassment by these white men, the only people she could go to were older white men. Would they side with her, a black woman, or with another white man? She wasn't going to risk her position in medical school to find out.

Decades later, there are still reports of women from all ethnic backgrounds who experience sexual harassment during their medical training yet never receive justice. The women have to find ways of coping with these painful experiences while maintaining the strength needed to succeed in medicine. Marilyn did just that: she tried to avoid or ignore the inappropriate jabs from her classmates and remain focused on her professional goals. When she reflected on that time, she wished she had had mentors who looked like her, who could have helped her navigate this difficult journey.[7] But there were only approximately ten black women and a hundred black men graduating from medical schools throughout the US in the ten years leading up to her own medical school graduation, and even fewer had been entering the field before then.[8] With such dismal numbers, Marilyn couldn't find a mentor who could relate to her struggles and help her navigate this ever-winding path.

After earning her medical degree, Dr. Marilyn Gaston (she had married by then) left Ohio briefly to complete her pediatric internship year at Philadelphia General Hospital. She strategically chose the hospital because it shared many of her values. As the first government-sponsored hospital in America dedicated to caring for the poor, it was a charity hospital that treated the sick and mentally ill while also providing housing and food for the homeless.[9]

On a chilly night, Dr. Gaston walked the halls of her new hospital. Although medical school had trained her for this next stage in her career, she was terrified. As a new doctor, she had learned much about the science behind disease, but she had precious little experience actually caring for patients. During that night, in the emergency room, Dr. Gaston strode briskly toward the room of her next patient. Abruptly, she came to a halt, struck by the piercing screams of a child on the other side of the door. She braced herself, then walked into the room. She was met by the sight of a baby boy with deep cocoa-brown skin. He was flailing incessantly. Then she saw it: his hand was red and swollen, as if someone had slammed it against a door. Alarms immediately sounded in Dr. Gaston's head.[10] This child was only six months old. He couldn't have injured himself. Who had hurt this baby?

Dr. Gaston hurriedly ordered tests, including an X-ray to confirm her suspicion of child abuse, and conducted a thorough physical exam. She was determined to protect this little boy. Whatever was needed, she did it. In the midst of this exhaustive workup, Dr. Gaston couldn't hold back her anger. She confronted the mother. "Something happened to this child. Who did this? Do you know who did this? How did this happen?"

Distressed, the mother quickly responded, "I don't know how it happened. It just happened! It just appeared!"

Unconvinced, Dr. Gaston resolved to admit the child to the hospital so that he could stay there until the abuser was revealed. She wanted to protect her patient from further abuse at home, even though she knew that admitting him with the suspicion of abuse could have serious repercussions for the family. Before Dr. Gaston could finalize this decision, her senior resident intervened. "Now, I hear you're admitting this baby," he said. He completed a thorough physical exam of the patient's hand and shook his head. "Marilyn, go look at a blood smear."[11]

Confused and embarrassed, Dr. Gaston ordered blood work on the child in order to analyze a blood smear. As she looked at the sample under the microscope, her heart stopped. Checkered among many normal-shaped red blood cells were multiple red blood cells with crescent moon shapes. They were sickled. Her face flushed with regret when she remembered accusing the poor mother of allowing her child to be abused. This baby wasn't a victim of abuse; he was suffering from sickle cell disease.

She hadn't learned much about sickle cell disease in medical school. Undoubtedly, the disease wasn't emphasized in school because sickle cell disease disproportionately affects people of African descent. There also wasn't a strong understanding of the biological mechanisms of sickle cell disease at the time, which may have further discouraged the school from including it in its curriculum. Regardless of the reasons, Dr. Gaston vowed to never make that mistake again. She knew the impact she had on her patients, and she recognized that her line of questioning and medical workup would likely become a traumatizing memory for the mother for years to come. Mistakenly admitting the child under suspicion of abuse could've broken up the family once social services got involved. Surely, she apologized profusely to the mother. But that wasn't enough. She vowed to dedicate her academic career to learning more about sickle cell disease. She hoped that through these efforts, sickle cell disease would never be mistaken for child abuse again.

Following her internship year, Dr. Gaston returned to Ohio, where she completed the rest of her pediatric residency at Cincinnati Children's Hospital Medical Center. When she was ready to enter the job market in the late 1960s, the landscape had changed dramatically from that of her predecessors. Dr. Gaston was in high demand. She was one of about fifteen black females, along with approximately a hundred black males, who graduated from an American medical school in 1964.[12] Thus, there were about 115 black physicians around the country looking for jobs at the same time as Dr. Gaston, following their residency training. In Cincinnati, only one African American pediatrician was already in practice. So, when Dr. Gaston began looking for job openings in Cincinnati, this African American female pediatrician sought to have Dr. Gaston join her private practice in order to have a greater impact in the black community. White physicians also sought to hire Dr. Gaston, seeing her as a shimmering token that would make their practice look more diverse and, thus, attract more patients.

The white practitioners' drive to hire black physicians reflected an immense cultural shift in America that began in the second half of the twentieth century. The civil rights movement had gained momentum in the 1950s. Second-wave feminism picked up steam just a decade later. Social pressure from these movements led to structural changes meant to address the intense race- and gender-based discrimination that had existed in the country for centuries. Passage of the landmark Civil Rights Act of 1964 and implementation of affirmative action policies gave women and black Americans access to educational and professional opportunities that they had been deprived of. Rejecting a medical school applicant or residency program applicant based on race or gender was no longer openly encouraged. While discrimination on those grounds persisted, it was oftentimes disguised as something else.

The movements and the legislation were meant to spur on gender and racial inclusivity in American society, but white men met this social pressure with the development of tokenism—a symbolic effort toward inclusion—rather than with actual inclusion. This tokenism particularly impacted the black community, allowing for the advancement of a few, while postponing, or even preventing, the advancement of the greater black community. The issue was discussed by many civil rights activists, including Malcolm X and Martin Luther King Jr.

In an interview with Louis Lomax in 1963, Malcolm X argued that, "in spite of all the dogs, and fire hoses, and club-swinging policemen," black people hadn't made any real gains. "All you have gotten is tokenism—one or two Negroes in a job or at a lunch counter so the rest of you will be quiet."[13] These inadequate changes were made, and then highly publicized, to quell the unrest in the black community that was amplified by the civil rights movement.

Martin Luther King Jr. echoed Malcolm X's discontent with tokenism in his book *Why We Can't Wait*, published in 1964. Dr. King explained that tokenism had been employed in the previous decade "to replace the old methods for thwarting the Negroes' dreams and aspirations."[14] Multiple large public schools in the South would allow a few black children to attend their schools, escorted by the US marshals to protect them from violent white townspeople. These few black students sprinkled among hundreds of white students were enough for the schools to declare themselves integrated. A major company would hire a single black employee and tout itself as being diverse. Dr. King argued that the limited number of black Americans who gained increased opportunities at that time were "tokens used to obscure the persisting reality of segregation and discrimination."[15] He went on to say that "those who argue in favor of tokenism point out that we must begin somewhere; that it is unwise to spurn any breakthrough, no matter how limited. . . . There is a critical distinction, however, between a modest start and tokenism. The tokenism Negroes condemn is recognizable because it is an end in itself. Its purpose is not to begin a process, but instead to end the process of protest and pressure. It is a hypocritical gesture, not a constructive first step."[16]

The interest that white physicians had in Dr. Gaston joining their medical practices represented one part of medicine's half-hearted attempts at integration. It must not be forgotten that she was one of only three African Americans out of four hundred students in the entire medical school student body. The medical institution created a bottleneck at the training level, severely limiting the number of black students who could enter. But the few who made it through (about 115 nationally in Dr. Gaston's graduation year) were rewarded with job opportunities. The presence of these few black physicians made it seem as though the medical profession was advancing toward racial equality, but the practice of tokenism kept true progress at a snail's pace.

D r. Gaston may not have thought much about the sociopolitical forces that spurred her job offers, but she still decided to turn them down. They didn't align with the commitment she still held from her childhood. The practices served primarily middle-class communities, and she wanted to care for patients from poor communities, people who experienced challenges similar to those her mother had faced as a result of limited access to healthcare. The primary route toward this goal was to work at community clinics. While her salary would be lower at a clinic than in private practice, she knew she would be paid dividends through her feeling of fulfillment. Initially, she rotated through a few Cincinnati Health Department clinics. She enjoyed the work, but deep down, she wanted more.

One day, Dolores J. Lindsay, a childhood friend, reached out to Dr. Gaston for help. Dolores, who had moved to the village of Lincoln

Heights, Ohio, about forty miles outside of Cincinnati, explained to her friend the dire situation her community was in. It was a very poor, African American area with limited access to healthcare. Many residents couldn't afford health insurance. Some didn't even have enough money to pay for the recommended vaccines. If a Lincoln Heights resident really needed to see a doctor, they had to go to Cincinnati or another big city just as far away. The high cost of transportation to distant locations was yet another hurdle. Dolores was tired of seeing her community suffer in this way. She implored Dr. Gaston to intervene. As Dolores spoke, Dr. Gaston likely felt bursts of excitement. This was the kind of work she had been looking for.

Dr. Gaston first dipped her toe into the water, testing out the temperature before fully diving in. She, along with a few other healthcare providers, volunteered their time to see if they could create an effective clinic. Dr. Gaston was the pediatrician. There was also an internal medicine doctor, a dentist, and a social worker. Once Dolores recruited all of the medical personnel, the team's members started to think about how they would acquire essential supplies for the clinic. They needed telephones, medications, needles, and more. First, they tried fundraising. Dolores went to the local American Medical Association chapter seeking financial support. Unmoved by her plea for support for the needy community, the chapter turned her away. She reached out to everyone else she could think of who might be willing to donate. They all said no; they didn't see her vision. Without benefactors, the clinic stood a slim chance of surviving.

But Dolores refused to give up. She had the idea of holding a press conference to show potential donors what she and the volunteers were doing. She refused to believe that people just didn't care about the plight of the community. They only needed to see it with their own eyes, so she made it happen. The volunteers scraped together any supplies that they could find in order to stock the clinic. Then, they invited community members who needed a healthcare visit to come by. A photographer captured pictures of the event.

One photo was so striking, it became impossible for people to turn their backs on the cause. A little boy sat on a cheap foldable chair in the middle of an empty court, located across the street from numerous worn buildings. Next to him stood a hunched Dr. Gaston as she tried to tune out external street sounds to listen to his heartbeat through her stethoscope. Simultaneously, she strained her eyes to examine him. The sole source of light was a loose-hanging lamp that fought against the dark of night closing in on the scene.

Journalists were so moved by this photo that it was placed, with an accompanying story, on the front page of the Cincinnati newspaper. Donations to the clinic started to pour in. With mounting community support, the clinic applied for and received a $10,000 grant from the Village of Lincoln Heights. Dolores Lindsay used this money, along with resources pooled from volunteer physicians and dentists, a handful of churches, and her own personal funds, to found the Lincoln Heights Health Center in October 1967. It was the first community health center in the state of Ohio.[17]

The center started in a four-room rented house on Matthews Drive. Confined to such a tight space, the volunteers learned to work like a well-oiled machine. The line of Lincoln Heights residents began at the door of the apartment and snaked around the block. Throughout each clinic day, the line was constantly replenished by more residents, who eagerly awaited a doctor's visit. For many, it would be their first in years. One by one, community members would enter the house and find Dolores on the first floor at the receptionist desk. Next to her would be a smiling three-year-old girl, the youngest of Dolores's five children. Each patient would be registered by Dolores. After providing a brief synopsis of the main issue that had brought them to the clinic that day, they would be directed upstairs.

On the second floor, the patient would find Dr. Gaston, who was so enamored with this project that she committed much of her time to working at the health center. The patient would also be met by other volunteer doctors and nurses stationed on the floor. They would be directed to a bedroom that had been converted into a patient exam room. The springboard beds that residents used to sleep on had been repurposed into exam room beds. When a patient needed to sit upright, the nurses would stack fluffy pillows against the bedframe to provide support for the patient's back. They could relax against the pillows as a doctor conducted a breast or stomach exam. All they had to do was lean forward off of the pillows when the doctor needed to press the smooth drum of their stethoscope against the thoracic portion of the patient's back to listen for the sound of the patient's lungs and check for signs of pneumonia and other lung diseases.

If the patient's chief complaint or medical history called for further tests, a nurse would collect blood or urine samples from the patient in the exam room and then take the samples down to the kitchen. This was the center's lab. A doctor would then prepare each sample and examine it under the microscope that sat on the kitchen table. The test results were important clues that helped the doctors come up with a diagnosis. Up the stairs the doctor would go, back to the second floor, where they would deliver a diagnosis to the patient. Together, the doctor and patient could then develop a treatment plan that would work within the patient's financial and/or lifestyle constraints, while also fulfilling their medical needs.

Once the doctor's visit was complete, a patient had the option to go to the basement, where they could receive a free dental exam. Some patients had teeth that were browning with decay because they had gone years without a dental exam. (An exam was just too expensive.) Now, the patients happily went to the basement to receive the dental care that they needed. The high-pitched dental drill must have seemed musical, promising meals free from toothaches. This community had wanted healthcare for years; now its members finally had that opportunity. In the first year, the doctors, dentists, and nurses served five hundred Lincoln Heights residents, more than 6 percent of the community's population.[18]

This health center still stands today, more than fifty years after its founding. It has moved from that small four-room apartment to a beautiful brown 42,000-square-foot building at the corner of Steffen and Mangham Avenues, about a fifteen-minute walk from the center's original location. Now referred to as the HealthCare Connection, the center has nine additional locations in nearby areas. Instead of a $10,000 grant and a handful of volunteers willing to give their time, the center works with an annual operating budget of $8.1 million and boasts ninety-five employees. In 2016 alone, this community health center conglomerate served 18,061 people with 44,409 visits.[19] Eighty-one-year-old Dolores Lindsay was still the organization's chief executive officer in 2017.

For Dr. Gaston, the community center provided her first lessons on developing community organizations. It solidified her passion for increasing access to quality care and improving health outcomes in underserved communities. Throughout her years of work in Lincoln Heights, Dr. Gaston maintained her connection with Children's Hospital Medical Center in Cincinnati. At various points in her service at the hospital, she met young patients experiencing the same splintering pain that the baby in Philadelphia endured. While this happened only a few years after she had graduated from medical school, her ability to recognize the signs of sickle cell disease had drastically improved. As Dr. Gaston worked up patients, sickle cell disease was at the top of her differential diagnosis. When she analyzed the blood smears under a microscope, she repeatedly spotted red blood cells shining back at her like crescent moons in the sky.

There was one patient with sickle cell disease. Then there were five. Then twelve. As Dr. Gaston discussed this upward trend with her colleagues, she crossed paths with Catherine Buford, a social worker who was seeing the same pattern. While considering their observations over lunch, they realized that they probably didn't understand the full scope of the issue. They wanted to know exactly how many sickle cell patients were being treated at the hospital. By organizing this information, they could figure out how to best serve the community. After rifling through a copious number of hospital charts, they tallied approximately eighty patients with sickle cell disease who had been treated at Cincinnati's Children's Hospital by 1969, only about four years after Dr. Gaston had started working at the hospital. Despite these increased numbers, whenever a patient received this diagnosis, the patient and the family felt alone in their experience.

Sickle cell disease has been heavily stigmatized because, as mentioned previously, it predominantly affects people of African descent, and its symptoms play into racist stereotypes. People with sickle cell disease regularly experience extreme pain when sickle-shaped red blood cells cluster together and obstruct blood flow to the chest, abdomen, or other parts of the body.[20] Opioids are needed to alleviate this pain. American medical institutions have historically provided limited funds to research the disease or to train physicians on how to care for patients. As a result, black patients would go to emergency rooms on a regular basis reporting extreme pain and requesting opioid medication. Their white physicians rarely believed that they were suffering from this pain—due to doctors' limited knowledge of the disease—and instead assumed that the black patients abused opioids and were lying about their symptoms to get their next fix.[21] Following the doctors' lead, school administrators and employers also didn't believe that this illness caused excruciating pain. So when sickle cell patients had to miss school or work due to painful sickle cell crises, they were viewed as lazy, instead of people in need of support as they weathered this difficult illness.[22] Due to the stigma, people who were impacted by the illness rarely talked about it. This silence prevented patients from recognizing the high prevalence of the disease.

Dr. Gaston and Ms. Buford saw their patients suffering both from the debilitating symptoms and the feeling of isolation, so they resolved to do something to help. Each patient and their family received an invitation to attend a sickle cell disease meeting at the hospital. The idea of publicly identifying with sickle cell disease likely made many feel vulnerable, somewhat akin to a person admitting that they were afflicted by AIDS at the height of the AIDS epidemic. Despite this, many patients and families showed up at the sickle cell conference. When they entered the room and saw so many other families, several were shocked. Dr. Gaston remembered family after family approaching her and Ms. Buford for confirmation: "All these children have sickle cell disease?"[23] The patients and families had felt so alone through their tormented journeys with the illness that it had seemed impossible that there were other people out there who understood what they were going through. Whenever a person asked Dr. Gaston and Ms. Buford this question, the doctor and the social worker would nod their heads in assurance. Soon the families were excitedly mingling with one another, finding comfort in their newfound community.

Dr. Gaston and Ms. Buford were so moved by the impact of the event, they started brainstorming ways to strengthen this new community. They started hosting regular meetings with the parents of the sickle cell patients. As the family members and healthcare providers sat side by side in a hospital meeting room, a reciprocal exchange took place. The families taught the healthcare providers what it was really like to live with this disease. With multiple families together, the providers were able to note shared experiences among the different patients and observe the unique ways the disease could manifest in an individual.

For the families, the meetings helped to give them strength on the days when they were sleep deprived because their child couldn't stop crying out in pain, or when the parents themselves were in tears as they thought about their child's poor prognosis. In the 1960s and 1970s, sickle cell patients typically didn't live past twenty years of age.[24] For this reason, the sickle cell meetings were composed mainly of the parents of sickle cell patients, not the patients themselves. Throughout their abridged lifetimes, these patients struggled with crippling pain and increased susceptibility to infections. Oftentimes, they lost their lives to multiorgan failure, or stroke, when obstruction of blood flow (from aggregation of their sickled red blood cells) became too severe. The patients and families needed a lot of emotional support to cope with the realities of the disease. For many, the meetings represented the first time that they had received this support from others who understood their struggle.

Because therapeutic options for sickle cell patients were so limited, Dr. Gaston and Ms. Buford started seeking government funding to research the disease. Their first stop was the Ohio state legislature, which had funds allocated for genetics research. Dr. Gaston and Ms. Buford knew that they wouldn't be successful if they embarked on the effort alone. At that time, very few people knew what sickle cell disease was. It would be difficult to convince a group of state legislators to invest in a mysterious disease. Instead, Dr. Gaston and Ms. Buford organized an event to raise awareness, leveraging the help of the parents and teenage sickle cell patients. One car followed another in a long caravan to the Ohio state capitol. The group requested a meeting with the director of the state health department. Once in front of her, the patients and families poured their hearts out, vulnerably sharing the anguish of living with the treacherous disease and having doctors who didn't have the answers to their questions about the illness. Dr. Gaston and Ms. Buford then made their case for how they could help the families if they were given adequate resources to do so. The health department director was shocked. She explained that she had never been asked for funds to tackle sickle cell disease. But she was moved by their presentation, so she gave them funding. Unfortunately, there was a limit to how much the director could give for sickle cell disease research because the state government had allocated most of the funds for research on genetic diseases to studies investigating cystic fibrosis. The funding that Dr. Gaston and her group received was enough to start some of their initiatives, but not enough to really study the mechanisms of or potential treatments for sickle cell disease. Expensive lab equipment and experimental reagents were over their budget.

This all changed on the frigid evening of February 18, 1971. As thousands of families huddled together in their living rooms to listen, President Richard Nixon proposed a new national health strategy.

> We often invest our medical resources as if an ounce of cure were worth a pound of prevention. . . . We focus our attention on making people well rather than keeping people well, and, as a result, both our health and our pocketbooks are poorer. A new National Health Strategy should assign a much higher priority to the work of prevention. . . . We must reaffirm—and expand—the Federal commitment to biomedical research. Our approach to research support should be balanced—with strong efforts in a variety of fields. Two critical areas, however, deserve special attention. The first of these is cancer. . . . A second targeted disease for concentrated research should be sickle cell anemia, a most serious childhood disease which almost always occurs in the black population. It is estimated that one out of every 500 black babies actually develops sickle cell disease. It is a sad and shameful fact that the causes of this disease have been largely neglected throughout our history. We cannot rewrite this record of neglect, but we can reverse it.[25]

President Nixon's new focus on sickle cell disease was likely influenced by increasing pressure from multiple civil rights organizations, including the Black Panther Party, as well as from other leaders in the black community at the tail end of the civil rights movement.[26] The collective silence from the government and medical community about sickle cell anemia became a prime example of the ways these institutions maintained practices that perpetuated racial health disparities. Public dissatisfaction had increased considerably in 1970, when Dr. Robert B. Scott published an article in the *Journal of the American Medical Association* documenting the scant funds allocated by the US National Institutes of Health (NIH) for sickle cell anemia research, as compared to funding for research on other genetic disorders such as cystic fibrosis, which primarily impacted white Americans.[27] Making sickle cell disease a priority allowed the Nixon administration to assert its concern for the black community at the same time it made other changes, like the dismantlement of the Office of Economy Opportunity (created to fight poverty in America), that hurt the community. Donna Spiegler, a staffer for Merlin DuVal, Nixon's assistant secretary of health and scientific affairs, even declared that the president's sickle cell anemia initiatives were "a gimmick for Nixon to get the black vote" during his second run for office.[28]

Regardless of his political motivations, President Nixon's decision to focus attention on sickle cell disease, through the allocation of $6 million for sickle cell disease research and initiatives, made a real impact. Dr. Gaston and Ms. Buford tapped into this funding via a grant from the NIH. Building upon their work funded by the state grant, they used the national funds to build a full-fledged sickle cell disease center.

Community centers became an essential tool for Dr. Gaston's public health endeavors. They gave community members the resources they needed to address the health disparities plaguing their own community. Because the healthcare providers were from the community, they understood the unique challenges other community members faced when trying to access healthcare. They understood their patients' beliefs around health and wellness, and even their fears in this arena. Any doctor could try to provide great care to their patients. But when the patients and doctors came from very different backgrounds, there was a lot that could be lost in translation. Dr. Gaston saw that community centers were a means to narrow this cultural divide. She poured herself into these community centers. She leveraged her experience at the Lincoln Heights Health Center to build the Sickle Cell Disease Center in Ohio. She was appointed director of the center in 1972 and served for four years. The center took a multifaceted approach to tackling sickle cell disease. It screened and diagnosed people, and it also conducted research on the disease and even held large educational programs about the condition. These services were so uncommon that the center received referrals for sickle cell patients from across the country.

In addition to making people aware of the disease and treating those who had been diagnosed, the center tried to tackle the psychological impact of being a patient or having a family member with sickle cell disease. Imagine having a child who was plagued by a disease that even doctors knew very little about. You would watch in terror as your child regularly cycled through crises that caused them to double over in crippling pain. You'd be flooded with a feeling of helplessness. Rushing to the ER would become a common ritual. During many of the visits, you and your child would have to sit in the waiting room for far too long. You would see multiple other patients receive attention ahead of your child. Was your family lower on the priority list because doctors didn't understand the severity of the pain your child was in, or was it because you all were black? You would try to stamp these questions out of your mind because the doctors were the only ones who could give your child some relief. You needed them. But still, treatment in the ER was only a flimsy Band-Aid for the problem. With each visit, dread would reverberate through your bones as you anticipated having to bury your child. The bleak prognosis of fewer than twenty years of life foretold the painful event. You would agonize at the thought that this would soon be your reality. Through it all, you would try to hide your own pain to be strong for your child.

Children with sickle cell disease live with this situation throughout their lives. They don't know any other way of life. Many of them likely sense the burden of fear and misguided sympathy countless unafflicted people place on them. They're people just like everyone else, but they're not always treated that way. Some people tiptoe around them, as if walking on eggshells. Others ostracize these children, as if they could catch the disease if the children got too close. The children show incredible resilience, but they're still suffering. How do you go through life with joy and hope when you're delivered a death sentence soon after birth? How do you dream about the future when every doctor tells you that you have none? As these children grow into adolescence, they understand their illness with increasing clarity. They're also more aware of what they'll miss out on due to their abridged lifespan. Someone in this position might find immense gratitude in the time they do have on earth, or they may fall into a deep depression as they process the gravity of their situation. Dr. Gaston's Sickle Cell Disease Center tried to lessen the emotional burden that these patients and families carried.

The center also tried to protect its patients' medical information. An easy genetic test was sufficient to diagnosis someone with sickle cell disease, so any entity with a person's genetic information would know with certainty when that person had been stricken with the disease. Health insurance companies sought this information so they could block sickle cell patients from acquiring health insurance; the companies didn't want to incur the medical costs of someone who wouldn't live long enough to pay them back with interest.

This discrimination was made even worse by society's poor understanding of sickle cell disease. It is an autosomal recessive disease, meaning that a patient with sickle cell disease has two copies of a mutated gene—one copy from each parent. Given the short lifespans of sickle cell disease patients in the 1980s, the people with the pertinent mutation who lived into their reproductive years were usually carriers of the sickle cell gene, not people with the disease.[29] They had only one copy of the mutated gene and were said to have sickle cell trait. People with sickle cell trait didn't have any symptoms, and they had normal lifespans. Many people with sickle cell trait never knew they had this mutation until screening for sickle cell disease became more prevalent. Screening was extremely important to help people with sickle cell disease, but it exposed people with sickle cell trait to the same prejudice that those with the disease experienced. People didn't understand the difference, so health insurance companies tried to prevent people with sickle cell trait from obtaining insurance. Recognizing this problem, the center had to think about how it would make this medical information accessible to other medical providers while safeguarding it from health insurance companies and other entities that sought to discriminate against people with one or two sickle cell genes. This was one of the first genetic diseases that faced this problem. The way this sickle cell health center, and others around the country, tackled the issue provided a blueprint for future work with other genetic diseases that subjected people to discrimination, particularly by health insurance companies.

Dr. Gaston enjoyed professional success and fulfillment at the Sickle Cell Disease Center, but she didn't stay. Her husband, Alonzo Gaston, received a job offer to teach at Howard University, so they moved to DC. While the move was motivated by his job, it ended up being a great opportunity for Dr. Marilyn Gaston as well. She was able to join the NIH, working as a medical expert in the Sickle Cell Center of the National Heart, Lung, and Blood Institute. She slowly rose up in the ranks, advancing to become deputy chief of the Sickle Cell Disease Branch and later serving as a member of the US Public Health Service Commissioned Corps in 1979.

She enjoyed the opportunity to work at the NIH, but her journey was not without its obstacles. Misogyny lurked in the shadows. One day, the issue came to light as Dr. Gaston was eating lunch with a male colleague. She had trained with him; both of them had completed pediatric residencies before working at the NIH together. They had the same job and even covered for each other when one was busy. He was her equal, but that was not how they were viewed.

Dr. Gaston remembered she had been taking a bite of food when her colleague casually said, "It was really nice to get that raise."

Her enjoyable meal was immediately soured. "I must've missed it."

Not realizing he had exposed the gender- and race-based inequity at their job, the colleague squirmed in his seat, suddenly regretting what he said. But Dr. Gaston wouldn't let it go. "Well, Omar, just tell me about the raise and how much it was."[30] Although he was hesitant at first, he eventually came clean: $20,000. This nonblack male physician had received $20,000 more than this black female physician to do the same job. Dr. Gaston was aware of identity-based wage gaps rampant within the workplace, but she refused to be a victim of this injustice.

Soon after this revelation, Dr. Gaston unapologetically strode into the office of the head of pediatrics to demand an answer. Dr. Gaston was unperturbed by the fact that the department head was a white man who might have given the selective raise due to prejudice. Once the director was available to talk with her, Dr. Gaston cut right to the chase. "I know Omar got a raise that I didn't. What's going on?"

"Don't take it personally. Your performance is wonderful, but Omar is supporting a family. He's a man. You have a husband."

Unwilling to back down, Dr. Gaston pushed the issue. "I don't understand. I am supporting a family too and he has a wife. So please help me with this connection." As her boss struggled to provide a reasonable, nonsexist explanation, she bravely made her stance clear. "I would like to get this straightened out as soon as possible or else I will have to—"[31] Before Dr. Gaston was able to outline her plan to report her boss's discriminatory actions, he promised to rectify the situation by giving her the same raise he had given her colleague. Addressing her boss's discriminatory actions could have gotten her fired. But Dr. Gaston refused to pour her talents into the organization unless she was treated fairly.

While Dr. Gaston was advocating for herself, she didn't lose sight of the people who had fallen victim to sickle cell disease. She leveraged the resources at the NIH to research some of the pressing questions she had about the disease. What was the clinical course of sickle cell disease, from a patient's birth to their death? How many people died from this disease? How accurate was the projected life expectancy? She started a huge study, partnering with medical institutions across the country, to tackle these difficult questions.

Dr. Gaston's clinical experience with sickle cell patients informed her research. She noticed a worrying trend of babies with sickle cell disease dying before they reached age four. For these children, the sharp edges of their sickle-shaped red blood cells damaged their spleens to the point of dysfunction. This left the children defenseless against life-threatening encapsulated bacteria, such as *Streptococcus pneumoniae* and *Neisseria meningitidis*. Dr. Gaston had witnessed tragic scenes of babies with sickle cell disease arriving at the ER with fever only to be declared dead less than nine hours later.

Because sickle cell screening was not in common practice, many of those babies had not even been diagnosed with sickle cell disease when they came in with severe infections. Doctors scrambled to figure out why a child was running a temperature, not realizing that the child was on a rapidly decreasing countdown toward death.

Dr. Gaston hypothesized that prophylactically treating young sickle cell patients with penicillin, an effective defense against many of the deadly infections in this patient population, could halt this deadly timer. But before doctors could give the vulnerable children this medication, they needed to know which children were at risk in the first place. This would require widespread screening for sickle cell disease. While there was general screening for other genetic diseases, like phenylketonuria (PKU) or hypothyroidism, many people were hesitant to implement screening for sickle cell disease. People with sickle cell disease or sickle cell trait were hesitant because they didn't want to become targets for discrimination, and geneticists were reluctant to screen because there was no treatment for sickle cell disease at the time. All doctors could do was treat the symptoms, such as the reoccurring pain. (It is common practice within the medical community to refrain from screening for incurable genetic diseases, because a diagnosis without any treatment can cause undue emotional harm to patients.)

Receptive to these concerns, Dr. Gaston led a landmark study on the efficacy of prophylactic penicillin treatment for babies with sickle cell disease. More than two hundred children with sickle cell disease, from multiple medical centers, were enlisted to participate in the study. The participants were randomly assigned to receive either oral penicillin or a placebo (like a sugar pill) twice daily. The assignments were double-blinded, meaning neither the participants nor the scientists knew which participant was receiving which medication. (This is a common research strategy to reduce bias that could skew the data.) Dr. Gaston and her team had to stop the trial eight months early, because the health outcomes were significantly different in the children receiving penicillin versus those with the placebo. There were fewer infections and deaths among the sickle cell children taking penicillin. Dr. Gaston's article on this study, "Prophylaxis with Oral Penicillin in Children with Sickle Cell Anemia," was the lead piece in the *New England Journal of Medicine* in 1986.[32]

With proof in hand, Dr. Gaston went to Capitol Hill to implore the government to create legislation that required newborn screening for sickle cell disease. It was a day that she would never forget. As she strode up the steps of the capitol building on a warm day in July, the sun shone on her face. Her nerves combined with the heat likely left her stomach queasy. As she faced rows and rows of white male politicians filling the House chamber, she tried not to feel intimidated. She drew her courage from her parents' teaching on the importance of believing in herself. The mantra from *The Little Engine That Could* rang in her mind, as it had at multiple other challenging points in her life: *I think I can, I think I can.* The words fueled her confidence as she delivered a compelling presentation to the governing body. Once Dr. Marilyn Gaston finished speaking, the government officials were convinced. Within three months, Congress had a bill to implement national screening for sickle cell disease. Two years later, forty states were screening babies for the disease.

Dr. Gaston had become such a leader within medicine that in 1990 she was appointed director of the Bureau of Primary Health Care, making her the first African American woman to lead a public health service bureau.[33] During her tenure, Dr. Gaston focused on strengthening health programs that catered to the unique needs of people who were poor or from otherwise disadvantaged backgrounds. She managed a $5 billion budget and served more than twelve million patients, including immigrants, people who were homeless, residents of public housing, and school-age children. By the time Dr. Gaston retired in 2001, she had reached the rank of assistant surgeon general. The job came with great responsibilities. Not many people could succeed as assistant surgeon general of the United States or in the various other leadership positions that she held. She had fulfilled her childhood determination to help make healthcare much more widely available, perhaps more significantly than even she had dared to dream.

But Dr. Marilyn Gaston believed that she could, so she did.

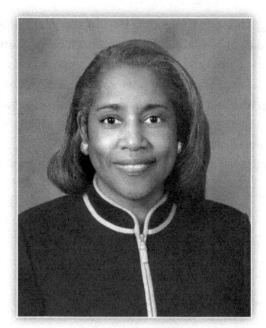

Dr. Claudia Thomas

"I WILL NOT BE THE LAST"

While the civil rights movement and second-wave feminism created immense societal pressure to make strides toward racial and gender equity in the 1950s and '60s, real progress was slowed by conciliatory measures, like giving a small number of black Americans and women access to various opportunities while maintaining oppression of the masses. This amounted to tokenism, which placated many members of these movements until civil rights leaders Malcolm X and Martin Luther King Jr. were assassinated, in 1965 and 1968, respectively. These events led to a resurgence in protests, putting more pressure on leaders in various fields to improve their efforts toward equity. Subsequently, more civil rights laws took effect, and white- and male-dominated institutions, including medical institutions, were forced to adhere to these new laws and those that preceded them.

An evolving physician workforce quickly emerged, one that included more white women and black Americans, and more people of color in general, throughout the country. The number of black women graduating from medical school each year leaped from about 25 in 1970 to about 700 in 2000.[1] The number of white female graduates increased from 1,714 in 1978 to 4,100 in 2000.[2] And between 1970 and 2000, the number of medical graduates from Indigenous American, Latinx, and Asian backgrounds increased fourteen-fold, fifteen-fold, and sixty-fold, respectively.[3] With increased representation came increased opportunities for these groups.

Sadly, one group's initial growth in medicine was quickly stifled by other, stronger social factors. The number of black male medical graduates was roughly 130 in 1970. This number quickly jumped to just under 450 in 1974.[4] But growth since that time has been almost nonexistent. The number of black male medical graduates dipped to 368 in 2015.[5] This is in contrast with all other POC groups, as well as white women, who have continued to grow in representation since the 1970s.

A major contributor to this sudden shift was the growth of mass incarceration. On June 17, 1971, President Richard Nixon delivered a speech to Congress on his goal of controlling high rates of illicit drug use. Nixon used strong rhetoric against illicit drug use, naming it "public enemy number one." Through the speech, the term "war on drugs" became popularized, and the country began to view its drug problem through a more militant lens. Following Nixon's encouragement, the government diligently pursued and imprisoned people suspected of selling drugs illegally, but it disproportionately targeted black men.[6] This led to a significant increase in incarceration levels, which was further exacerbated by the actions of President Ronald Reagan's administration. From Reagan's election in 1980 to the election of his successor, George H. W. Bush, in 1988, the US prison population nearly doubled, from 329,000 to 627,000.[7] To this day, the US holds a larger prison population than any other nation in the world, including China, which has a population that exceeds the US population by over one billion people.[8] And black Americans, particularly black men in America, are disproportionately impacted by this often for-profit bondage system.

So many black boys are absorbed into the criminal system. All it takes is a minor mistake, like the one made by the little boy in Dr. Ferebee's neighborhood who was just trying to feed his baby brother. Or, too commonly, a black man can be imprisoned for a crime he did not commit. Once he is locked in that cage, any chance of a prosperous future, especially one in professions like law or medicine, vanishes.

It is impossible not to compare the black man's plight to the black woman's. Black men had the upper hand in medicine from the moment Dr. James McCune Smith entered the field in 1837. For 150 years, black men outnumbered black women in medicine. But in 1988, this trend switched. The number of black women entering medicine exceeds that of black men today, though black women are still severely underrepresented within medicine, making up only 2 percent of the physician workforce in 2020.[9] Still, we cry out for the injustice we see perpetuated against our black brothers. From 1990 to 2011, the gap between the number of black women and the number of black men in medical schools widened dramatically, from 5 percent to 43 percent.[10] Despite this startling national trend, I am fortunate to have a black medical class that's almost evenly split. There are nearly 170 students in my class, 23 of whom are black: 10 black women and 13 black men. But some medical classes are significantly lopsided. A recent medical school class with a size similar to mine had about 20 black students but only 3 black men. This is a dire situation that both black men and black women physicians are trying to address.

Claudia Thomas was born in Brooklyn, New York, in 1950 amid this changing climate. Neither of her parents, Charles and Daisy Thomas, had the opportunity to receive a college education, so they poured their hopes and aspirations into Claudia and her older sister, Catharine. Charles provided financial support for the family by working long hours as a truck driver, while Daisy stayed at home and invested countless hours helping her daughters develop their minds.

Daisy transformed her kitchen table into a school desk, where she tutored her daughters on key concepts that would help them succeed once they started formal schooling. One learning tool she used was a wooden scale that resembled a toy. A person would place two blocks on one scale and one block on the other. Voilá! It balanced! The blocks had different sizes, but the most salient feature of each was a number that shone on the block face. Eventually, Claudia started to notice a pattern. The seven block was on the left scale. The three and four blocks on the right. Over and over, she would try different combinations on the scales. She memorized which combination of blocks balanced each other and, by extension, which numbers she had to add together to equal a specific value. It was simple addition. With their mother's support, Claudia and Catharine also learned subtraction and the alphabet, and how to sign their names—all before they entered kindergarten.

Daisy remained involved in Claudia's education when Claudia started school. Daisy joined the Parent Teacher Association and volunteered at the school so that she could stay informed about what was going on. One day, Claudia's teacher gave her a B when she had earned an A. The teacher's rationale: it was too early in the semester to give Claudia an A. Well, it didn't take long for this incident to get back to Daisy. Immediately, she was in that teacher's office demanding that the teacher give her child the grade she deserved. Charles's long work hours made it difficult for him to advocate the way his wife did. But he also made it known that he wanted his daughters to excel in school.

During Claudia's early years, the educational system underwent a significant overhaul. The *Brown v. Board of Education* Supreme Court case was decided when she was four years old. Some white school administrators anticipated the reversal of the 1896 *Plessy v. Ferguson* Supreme Court decision. Without racial segregation of schools, they had to do something to maintain white supremacy. A year before the *Brown v. Board* ruling, Darla Buchanan, a black teacher in Topeka, Kansas, received a letter from Wendell Godwin, the city's superintendent. It read: "[T]he majority of people in Topeka will not want to employ Negro teachers next year for white children. It is necessary for me to notify you now that your services will not be needed for next year."[11]

Darla was among teachers affected by the early wave of black teacher layoffs. Once the Supreme Court decision was finalized, white superintendents fired tens of thousands of black teachers and principals. The representation of black educators nosedived, from between 35 and 50 percent in the seventeen states that had segregated school systems to about 7 percent of public school teachers today.[12] Numerous black teachers were highly qualified, with PhDs and years of teaching experience. But they lost their jobs because black teachers and principals couldn't hold positions of intellectual authority over young white students. This would challenge the myth that white people are smarter than black people. The number of black teachers has yet to rebound since this Supreme Court decision.[13] Though *Brown v. Board* allowed black kids, like Claudia, to have access to more well-resourced schools, it also deprived them of black educators, who were typically more supportive of black children and, of course, served as role models.

Many white educators, including some of Claudia's, had lower expectations for their black students. They believed that the potential success of a black person could be determined when they were still a child. In a 2011 interview, Claudia remembered when she was in first or second grade and her teachers made her take a test that she wasn't supposed to tell her parents about. The test, like many others being used around the country, was used to separate the "smart" kids from the "dumb" kids. But these tests were biased against the black children.[14] The teachers administering these tests wanted to use a measure purported as objective to perpetuate their racist views. The children who struggled on the test were placed in slower-paced classes, while the children who performed well were placed in the faster-paced classes. Because the test was designed to advantage the white children, white children made up the majority of the advanced classes, while black children made up a large proportion of the slower classes. This led to an educational gap that grew wider each year. Eventually, this chasm would be too great to overcome. And neither the black children, nor their parents, would understand why. Thankfully, Claudia's teachers' attempts to sabotage her academic progress were unsuccessful, due to the extra lessons her mother gave her outside of school, combined with the encouragement from both of her parents to pursue academic excellence.

When Claudia entered sixth grade, the Open Enrollment Act was passed in New York. It aimed to reduce racial segregation in schools by allowing students to attend any public school in the state regardless of their district of residency.[15] Following the Brown v. Board of Education decision, racial segregation of schools was maintained through racial segregation of neighborhoods, i.e., redlining. This act allowed Claudia to attend a more well-resourced, predominantly white junior high school in Kew Gardens, Queens, which she would need to take a bus and multiple subway lines to reach.

At this school, she saw the consequences of the biased tests that had been administered in her early years of primary school. Claudia was in the advanced classes, oftentimes as the only black student in the room. But when she walked the hallways, she saw the slow-paced classes packed with black students. This racial stratification of students hadn't been as obvious when she attended predominantly black schools.

Claudia's experience elicits memories of my own childhood. It was the same dynamic in school, more than fifty years later. I was almost always the only black student in my Advanced Placement classes, while most of the black students at my school were in the average- or slow-paced classes. This never made sense to me, because many of my black friends were just as smart as me. But I didn't understand the larger system. I had moved to New Jersey in eighth grade, a transplant into the community.

I had been in advanced math classes leading up to that point and was positioned to start in advanced geometry. But my new school tried to move me back two levels, to regular algebra. My parents had to advocate on my behalf. They convinced the school to allow me to take a qualification exam for the two-year advanced geometry course. I passed. That advanced geometry class set me up for more advanced math and science classes in high school. After seeing parallels to Claudia's story, I wondered if race had anything to do with my own experience.

If I was not black, would my parents have had to work as hard to keep me on track? Were my black classmates victims of a racial education gap introduced by the educational institution? Or are the similar racial dynamics at my high school and Claudia's just a coincidence? I felt so supported by my middle school and high school. I would feel gutted if they were involved in stifling the educational development of my black peers.

Even though Claudia struggled with the social dynamics of school, her family kept her grounded. With their continuous support, Claudia performed well at the High School of Music and Art in New York City.[16] She even qualified for the National Merit Scholarship, based on her exceptional academic record and high scores on national scholastic aptitude examinations.[17] She also qualified for the competitive New York State Regents Scholarship.[18] These scholarships helped her pay for tuition at Vassar College, a liberal arts college about two hours from her home. This college experience was defining for Claudia. She stated simply: "I found out who I was at Vassar . . . as an African American."[19]

Claudia arrived on her college campus in the fall of 1967 as a bright-eyed seventeen-year-old. She had just gotten her hair done. Her locks glistened in the sun and flowed down her back. She was confident. Like many college freshmen, she wanted to reinvent herself. She wasn't really aware of what was happening in the broader black community or in the civil rights movement. She was a free black girl, enjoying the apparent simplicity of her life. This all ended in the spring of her first year. Her world view changed profoundly on the night of April 4, 1968, when Martin Luther King Jr. was assassinated.

For many days after that, Claudia was in mourning. She felt as if a hole had been carved out of her heart. This response seemed natural. Instinctive. So she was shocked when she realized her white classmates hadn't responded in the same way. So many of them seemed unfazed by the loss of this iconic changemaker. This is when Claudia realized that they were different. They lived in separate worlds. This was the beginning of her journey toward understanding the complex dynamics of race in America.

Her altered perspective impacted the way she moved in the world. Instead of the straight locks she came to school with, she started rocking her natural hair. The increasing size of her Afro signified her burgeoning black pride. She helped create, and then lead, Vassar's Students' Afro-American Society. Conversations with members of this organization helped her solidify her stance on racial issues perpetuated by her college. The number of African American students and professors was far too small. The school needed to be more representative of the American population. The American history program focused almost exclusively on the experience of white Americans. It was time the school established a black studies program. So many American universities were built on the backs of African Americans, but so few deemed it necessary to provide a curriculum that included teachings on the African American experience.

Claudia was tired of the injustice. She partnered with some of her black classmates and, together, they went to the faculty to advocate for these changes. When their requests fell on deaf ears, they followed the example of the late Martin Luther King Jr. and organized peaceful protests. In October 1969, members of the Afro-American Society staged a sit-in at Vassar's main building for four days. They slept there and ate there, and they refused to return to classes until the administration listened to their concerns and took action. It wasn't until the sit-in gained national attention that the school responded—it wanted to minimize the negative press. Vassar agreed to establish a black studies major and committed to make efforts to increase the number of black students and professors.[20]

For most of Claudia's time at Vassar, she studied mathematics. But by her junior year, she became concerned about her trajectory. Her higher-level classes were increasingly theoretical. She was most interested in applied mathematics, particularly geometry. She also realized that a math degree would pigeonhole her into a career as either a math teacher or math theorist. Neither of these appealed to her. Through the process of elimination, she eventually decided to pursue a career in medicine. As a doctor, she could help people through the field of biology, which had been an interest of hers since high school.

Vassar didn't have a premed major at the time, so she just switched her major from mathematics to black studies. She conducted a sickle cell anemia project in which she analyzed the blood samples of over two hundred residents of Poughkeepsie, New York, following in the footsteps of a woman she didn't yet know to admire. Claudia wanted to determine if they had the sickled blood cell deformity. Her work was notable enough to have been published in a scientific journal. In addition to this project, she needed to complete her premed requirements. She had already taken math, physics, and foreign languages. She jampacked the remaining biology and chemistry courses into her schedule in her senior year and began applying to medical school. By the spring, she received the wonderful news that she had been accepted into Johns Hopkins University School of Medicine.

When she first started medical school in 1971, she was blown away. The demands of her previous schools were nothing in comparison to those of medical school. If you fell behind a little bit, it was an uphill battle to get back on track. While she was in medical school, "missing a day of class [meant] missing thirty chapters of reading."[21] To progress through school, Claudia had to work diligently and adapt to the new environment.

This classroom-style learning lasted only for the first two years. Once she learned the theory, it was time to apply it. Claudia was shipped off to the hospital, where she rotated through multiple core specialties, including internal medicine and surgery. This experience helped her develop her clinical skills while exploring different career paths. Would she do pediatrics? How about psychiatry? Figuring out which specialty she would pursue was a process.

The first step was deciding if she wanted to do medicine or surgery. Claudia considered her nonclinical passions when making her selection. She had loved art since she was a young girl. While she didn't want to pursue a career as a professional artist, she held on to her creativity. Claudia also had extensive experience sewing. She learned this skill from her mother, who worked as a seamstress. Years with the sewing needle taught Claudia dexterity. She believed these two skills would aid her in surgeries.

Once Claudia decided that she wanted to be a surgeon, she had to figure out what kind. The general surgeons she worked with during her clerkship year made her wary of that specialty. Many of them were angered too easily. When one got angry, the entire operating room became uncomfortable. When stress was high, some surgeons took their frustrations out on other members of the care team. They would curse at the nurses or throw instruments. Claudia didn't want to be around this negative energy.

As Claudia contemplated her other options, she passed a huge statue of Christ positioned in the main rotunda of the Johns Hopkins Hospital.

Although she had seen it before, she looked in awe at the sandy-gray Italian marble statue. It made her imagine sculpting the human body. Intrigued by this prospect, she investigated plastic surgery. While she was exploring this path, she attended an orthopedic lecture at the school. Suddenly, it all clicked. She could reshape the human body by helping broken bones heal correctly. She could help people who were plagued by malformed bones. This specialty combined the carpentry skills that her father had taught her and the sewing skills that she learned from her mother, and her artistic mind.

Toward the end of Claudia's medical school career, she knew she wanted to be an orthopedic surgeon. She just wasn't sure how she would fit into the space. She confided in her chief resident: "You know, I like this stuff. It's really catching on. But I don't see any women doing orthopedic surgery."[22] She would later find out that there were only twenty-five women out of approximately ten thousand orthopedic surgeons nationally, none of whom were African American.[23]

Without hesitation, Claudia's resident turned to her and said assuredly, "There's no reason that you can't do this."[24] Her worries immediately disappeared. That was all the encouragement she needed.

While in the wards, Claudia saw more than just surgeries. Johns Hopkins Hospital, like every other predominantly white hospital in the US, racially segregated its patients throughout most of the twentieth century. This not only affected where a "white" or "colored" patient received care; it affected the kind of care they received. The "colored" wards at Johns Hopkins opened in March 1894. They were dilapidated in comparison to the "white" wards. Even the patient samples were stored differently. There were shelves labeled "white blood" and "colored blood," each containing matching blood bottles that either said "white" or "colored."[25]

These ever-present distinctions facilitated bias in the clinical practice at the time. If a fridge filled with tissue samples had a power outage, it would be natural for a white medical professional to save the "white samples" before they went to rescue the "colored samples." This could compromise the integrity of those "colored samples," which could lead to an inaccurate diagnosis and an ineffective, or even harmful, treatment regimen for those black patients.

As societal norms around race relations changed, policy followed. At Hopkins, the hospital wards slowly began to desegregate in 1959, with the surgery department first to make the change. Some wards, like the psychiatry department, maintained this racist practice for longer. The hospital wasn't fully desegregated until 1973, two years after Claudia started medical school.

When Claudia rotated through a ward that integrated in 1964, she felt like the physicians and nurses had not yet adjusted to the change. She explained: "I would hear things that displeased me, insulted me."[26] There was a time when a seventy-year-old man was transferring from his hospital bed to a stretcher. Maybe he was about to undergo a surgery. During this transfer process, a young white resident proclaimed, "Atta boy, atta boy."[27] Despite being almost fifty years younger than the patient, this resident felt comfortable calling this patient a boy.

There is a long history of white people referring to black men and women as "boys" and "girls." It was a tactic used to belittle and demoralize this community. Claudia was already exhausted by the intense demands of medical school. There's no telling how many hours she had spent in the hospital the week that this incident happened. But when she witnessed this racist encounter, she felt compelled to speak up. She turned to the resident and said, "I'm sorry. I don't know how you consider yourself. But this is a man, and I would appreciate if you would address this person with the respect that's due."[28]

When Claudia challenged her supervising resident on their behavior, she made herself extremely vulnerable. Medical students' grades in their clinical rotations are based on their residents' and attendings' subjective views of their performance in the wards. This resident's behavior suggested that they had prejudice against black people, which likely negatively impacted their assessment of black medical students' performance in the hospital. Claudia's decision to advocate for her black patient could have motivated this resident to give her an even more detrimental assessment. It could have had negative repercussions on her career.

Following this encounter and others like it, Claudia's white colleagues ostracized her. They tried to gaslight her, claiming that their racist behavior wasn't prejudiced. She was tagged as "seeing a racist behind every tree."[29] But she wasn't delusional. She wasn't overreacting. The difference in medical care for their white patients versus their black patients was palpable.

Despite this injustice, Claudia's advocacy for her black patients could prevent her from graduating from medical school. It distracted her from her school obligations, such as giving clinical presentations in the wards or performing well on exams after each rotation. It would be easier if she had acted like many of her white classmates, who turned a blind eye to the racial injustice. But she couldn't do that. She decided to add patient advocacy to her long list of responsibilities. Thankfully, this heavy burden didn't cause her to burn out. She completed all her medical school requirements and graduated from Johns Hopkins University School of Medicine in the spring of 1975. A few weeks later, Dr. Claudia Thomas joined Yale New Haven Hospital as a new orthopedic surgery intern.

Interns are newly minted doctors who are still relatively low on the totem pole. Many in this position opt to keep their heads down and try not to ruffle any feathers. But, as in medical school, Dr. Thomas chose not to take this easy path. When she saw problems in the hospital, she voiced her concerns. One of her more memorable experiences during her intern year occurred when she was working with a neurosurgeon whose attitude rivaled that of the general surgeons that she had encountered in medical school. While neurosurgery cases can be extremely stressful, this surgeon didn't manage his stress in a productive way. He liked to take his stress out on the women on his care team, including Dr. Thomas.

Dr. Thomas was performing a surgery with this physician, and, at one point, she did something that he didn't like. Immediately, he aimed his aggression at her. "You're so g-ddamn stupid!"[30] She felt completely disrespected, but she tried to smooth over the tension by explaining her choice of actions. He didn't want to hear it. He just kept cursing at her. Dr. Thomas's blood began to boil as this man's sexist behavior weighed more heavily on her. He never treated the men this way. Dr. Thomas decided that she would not take this man's assault. She tore off her gown and gloves and stormed out of the OR. This response was bold. While the neurosurgeon was the one engaging in verbal harassment, Dr. Thomas was a lowly intern. She was the one who broke the norms of medicine by speaking out against her superior. Her livelihood was now at risk. The neurosurgeon knew the power he held in the situation, so he tried to get Dr. Thomas fired. Luckily, the residency director did not give in to his request. Dr. Thomas was allowed to stay and complete her residency.

As she continued through her training, the number of surgeons who respected and supported her professional development outnumbered those who tried to throw barriers in her way or demean her. This mentorship was vital to Dr. Thomas's advancement. Still, she faced a challenge that was unique to being a woman. She had chosen orthopedic surgery, a physically demanding specialty. Orthopedic surgeons commonly work with joints that are difficult to maneuver, including the hip, the largest joint in the body. To put a dislocated hip back into place requires sheer force, and there aren't machines to assist in this endeavor. Success sometimes depends on the strength of the surgeon, which explains why many of the men who entered this field were athletes. Dr. Thomas did not fit this mold. But she was not deterred. She found a way to adapt. She couldn't use the techniques that the men used to maneuver a dislocated hip, so she developed one of her own.

One day, she was scrubbing in with a Dr. Keggi, a strong Nordic orthopedic surgeon. As Dr. Thomas looked on, Dr. Keggi removed the patient's dislocated hip with ease. Now, it was time to put the new prosthetic hip into place. Dr. Keggi was comfortable with this procedure; he had completed countless hip replacement cases. He began his tugging and pulling to put the hip in. But the prosthetic wouldn't give. He applied more force. Still, no progress. The scrub nurse gave the patient a relaxant so that the muscles would be more pliant. Dr. Keggi used all of his strength, but it just wouldn't budge. The prosthetic must have been too long. Resigned, Dr. Keggi lumbered to the back table to pick out another one. There was a whole process involved in replacing the current prosthetic with a new one. This would take hours.

Dr. Thomas surveyed the room; besides Dr. Keggi, everyone in the room was a woman. She confidently turned to the anesthesiologist, ready to take charge. "Give the patient some more relaxant."[31] Then, she motioned to a scrub nurse and asked her to hold the patient down. Dr. Thomas used her unique technique to drive the prosthetic hip into place. There was a satisfying "pop" that confirmed her success.

After five long years of a challenging but rewarding residency, Dr. Claudia Thomas completed the program in 1980. She was the first woman graduate of Yale's orthopedic residency program and the first black woman orthopedic surgeon in the country.[32] Dr. Thomas was not herself impressed by this distinction. Instead she said, "When I learned that I was the first African American female orthopedic surgeon, I said, Well, I will not be the last."[33] As in her days at Vassar, she was committed to bringing others up as she climbed. And she did just that.

After completing her residency and a brief fellowship in shock trauma, Dr. Thomas was appointed assistant professor of orthopedic surgery at the Johns Hopkins University School of Medicine. She used her privileged position as a faculty member to support others. Over the course of her tenure, Dr. Thomas helped recruit a high number of underrepresented minorities and women to train in orthopedics at Johns Hopkins. When she joined the faculty in 1981, the orthopedic residency program had trained only one woman and one black man in its history. By 2008, 20 percent of Hopkins's orthopedic residency class were women and 32 percent were black.[34]

Dr. Jamil Jacobs-El, a former Hopkins orthopedic surgery resident from the class of 1995, described the impact Dr. Thomas had on his life: "It is very possible that I would not be a practicing academic orthopedic surgeon today, nor have as many superbly trained colleagues if it were not for Dr. Thomas' valiant and selfless efforts on our behalf. Dr. Thomas represents a rare and necessary entity to advance the cause of orthopedic surgery training, beyond the scope of her own private practice, with a vision to the future of medicine."[35]

The 2007 president of the American Academy of Orthopaedic Surgeons (AAOS), Dr. James Beaty, also sang Dr. Thomas's praises: "She was determined to help minority women enter orthopaedics and has been responsible for scores of minorities and women entering our profession. Dr. Thomas has provided orthopaedic care to inner city residents and has encouraged colleagues and protégés to do exactly the same. For the past 30 years, her tenacity and social activism have been responsible for extraordinarily diverse residency programs in institutions across the country."[36] Dr. Thomas's avid mentorship and advocacy work led to her receiving the AAOS Diversity Award in 2008.

Dr. Thomas's dedication to mentorship inspired some of her mentees to become impactful mentors themselves. One such mentee was Dr. Bonnie Mason. When Dr. Mason was in medical school, she shared her dreams of becoming an orthopedic surgeon with a trusted advisor. Their response was, "You will NEVER be an orthopedic surgeon as a little black girl from a little black school."[37] These words were painful and discouraging, but meeting Dr. Thomas not too long after this encounter reaffirmed Dr. Mason's conviction to pursue orthopedics.

Dr. Mason's feelings from her first meeting with Dr. Thomas mirror those of Dr. Joycelyn Elders when she first met Dr. Edith Irby Jones. Dr. Mason recalled, "Well, the first time I laid eyes on Dr. Claudia Thomas, the first African-American woman to become a board-certified orthopedic surgeon in the U.S., I knew I could do it. In my mind, she looked just like me, which underscores the power of our presence. . . . Dr. Thomas was one of my first mentors in orthopedics and remains so to this day. Her strength, courage and achievements continue to inspire me."[38] In 2004, only four years after completing her orthopedic surgery residency at Howard University, Dr. Mason founded Nth Dimensions, a mentoring program aimed at addressing the dearth of women and underrepresented minorities in orthopedic surgery while eliminating healthcare disparities for all communities.[39] Since its founding, Nth Dimensions has awarded over $1.2 million in scholarships and program grants while exposing thousands of students to the field of orthopedic surgery.[40]

The unwavering efforts of Dr. Thomas and Dr. Mason were necessary in a field that has been resistant to change. In 2019, orthopedic surgery was the least diverse field out of all medical and surgical subspecialties. In recent years, approximately 50 percent of all US medical school graduates have been women. Despite this, only 14 percent of orthopedic surgery residents are women. Worse still, black and Latinx trainees make up only 4.1 percent and 2.7 percent of all orthopedic residents, respectively.[41] The well-documented scarcity of women and racial minorities in surgical subspecialties is intensified in orthopedic surgery. Without the strong mentorship and advocacy employed by Drs. Claudia Thomas and Bonnie Mason, the demographic of orthopedic surgeons would be even more lopsided—maintaining a near-complete domination of the field by white male orthopedic surgeons through the exclusion of those from other genders and racial backgrounds.

One thing that deters many women from pursuing orthopedic surgery, and many other surgical subspecialties, is the extremely demanding nature of their residency training programs, which makes it difficult to have a family. When Dr. Thomas was in her residency program, she left home for the hospital at six in the morning and didn't return until around ten at night. Her time was not her own. Even though she wanted to have a family, she felt compelled to put it off. She committed herself to the surgical training process throughout her residency and fellowship. But once she became an attending physician, at thirty-one years old, she jumped into the dating scene.

Unfortunately, she struggled to find a partner who supported her career. Her potential suitors didn't value her work as a trailblazing orthopedic surgeon. They saw orthopedics as a distraction that would take her away from her true womanly duties. These men expected Dr. Thomas to prioritize cooking and cleaning, and even doing their laundry. Norms around which partner in a heterosexual relationship should make the most money posed another challenge that she, and many female physicians, faced. Dr. Thomas dated a city councilman who once commented, "I could make $100,000, but I still wouldn't make as much as you."[42] Dr. Thomas knew that her earning potential far outpaced that of many working men. She was comfortable with that. She didn't believe that a man's masculinity, or his potential to be a good partner, was dependent on whether he was the highest earner in the household. But this man couldn't get past Dr. Thomas's success. He became so insecure that the relationship fell apart.

Fortunately, Claudia eventually met Maxwell Carty, a man who loved her and appreciated all that she had to offer.[43] They married in 1985, when Claudia was thirty-five. Her husband was not an orthopedic surgeon; he was a builder. Maxwell could have worried that Claudia would command more respect than he did, due to her profession, but he was secure within himself. He didn't tie his masculinity to his ability to dominate his wife. And he didn't try to hold her back. He was proud of all that Dr. Thomas had achieved and supported her career as a loving partner should.

Once Claudia and Maxwell got settled in their marriage, they tried to have kids. By this point, Claudia was around forty years old. Due to a markedly reduced number of healthy eggs and the immense physical toll that a pregnancy has on a woman's body, having a baby becomes particularly difficult for women in their mid- to late thirties. Claudia was forced to accept the heartbreaking reality that her dream of having children would never be realized—her career and life course up to that point had rendered this impossible. One way that she coped with this loss was by pouring her love into many young medical trainees, several of whom were aspiring orthopedic surgeons.

The residency training for orthopedic surgery, and for many other medical and surgical subspecialties, was designed for men. Its grueling hours serve to ward off any woman audacious enough to consider joining this exclusive community. Either they give up their aspirations of becoming a physician, or they risk not being able to have children. Dr. Thomas tried to have both, and experienced agony when she couldn't have children due to a system that was stacked against her.

A more heterogenous workforce in orthopedic surgery, and medicine as a whole, allowed women and underrepresented minorities to get involved in decisions around residency training, which led to the establishment of more inclusive policies. When Dr. Thomas was a trainee, it was normal for residents to work as much as 120 of the 168 hours in the week at the hospital. In 2003, the Accreditation Council for Graduate Medical Education (ACGME) enacted "duty hour" restrictions, capping the average work hours for a resident to eighty hours a week.[44] While residents in various specialties still report working more than eighty hours a week, residents generally work fewer hours than their predecessors.[45] Diversity efforts from people like Dr. Claudia Thomas were essential to alter the work culture of medicine, making it more feasible for people to pursue this profession without making significant sacrifices in their personal lives. Thanks to Dr. Thomas's tireless commitment to increasing professional opportunities and improving the work environment for women and people of color, it's more feasible for someone like me to become a surgeon.

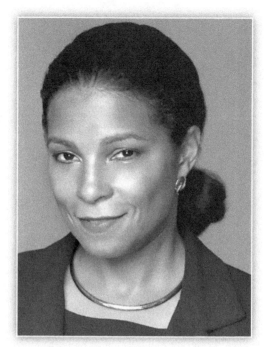

Dr. Risa Lavizzo-Mourey

CHAPTER 9

CRUSADING FOR PUBLIC HEALTH

N owadays, the path to medicine begins the same way for everyone—
we attain an undergraduate degree, complete our required premed
classes, and take the MCAT, which is the national standardized medical
school admissions test. A student can come from almost any college or
university in the US and still be competitive for most medical schools.
They just need to have strong GPAs and MCAT scores and take the prerequisite courses in college, participate in extracurriculars, and exhibit
a passion for medicine.

But as soon as the student receives admission into one or more medical schools, that path toward medicine splinters into a dozen distinct
directions. The student could attend an allopathic or osteopathic medical school, leading to an MD or DO, respectively. They could choose a
medical school located in the mainland US or the Caribbean islands, or
even further abroad. They could pick the more expensive school or the
school with the best financial aid. Many aspiring physicians are in their
early twenties when they make this crucial decision, which can impact
what medical specialty they go into or if they can afford to buy a house
in their thirties. Since I will be the first person in my family to become
a doctor, I didn't have a built-in support system to guide me along this
convoluted path.

To make matters more complicated, I am a black woman with aspirations of making a significant impact in medicine. I've dreamt of
being selected for top leadership positions in medicine, such as dean
of a medical school. But when I researched who held these positions, I
found that it was still overwhelmingly men. According to the Association of American Medical Colleges, in 1991, 100 percent of all permanent

medical school deans were men. This position has become only a little more inclusive over the years. In 2020, 82 percent of all permanent medical school deans were men.[1] And despite searching for over a year, I've been able to find only two black women who are currently deans of medical schools: Dr. Valerie Montgomery Rice and Dr. Deborah Prothrow-Stith.[2] They lead two of the four historically black medical schools, Morehouse School of Medicine and Charles R. Drew University of Medicine and Science, respectively. What did they, and other black female leaders in medicine, have to do to attain positions that allowed them to have wide-reaching impacts in medicine? How did they combat the race- and gender-based prejudice that likely impacted other people's perceptions of these black women's ability to lead?

As these questions swarmed in my mind, I stumbled upon an interview with Dr. Risa Lavizzo-Mourey. This black woman physician is a global leader and a professor at my school, the University of Pennsylvania. I promptly reached out to her since we shared this institutional connection. Like the reaction Dr. Joycelyn Elders had when she first met Dr. Edith Irby Jones, I buzzed with excitement and hope after meeting Dr. Lavizzo-Mourey. Learning about her journey made me believe that my dreams of positively impacting medicine, particularly by making the medical profession more inclusive and by reducing health inequities, are actually things that I can achieve. Lessons from her past, and from those of every other black woman physician in this book, light the way for my future.

Risa Lavizzo was born in Nashville, Tennessee, in 1954, four years after Claudia Thomas was born. Risa was raised by parents who had both managed to become physicians. Her mother, Dr. Blanche Sellers Lavizzo, was a pediatrician, and her father, Dr. Philip Lavizzo, was a surgeon. Before the couple had any children, they spent a year in Seattle, Washington, while Philip completed his surgical residency. After, the couple returned to Nashville to begin their medical practices.

Soon after Risa was born, the Lavizzos received better job opportunities in Seattle and decided to move back permanently. This move allowed them to raise their children outside the Jim Crow South. Although the Lavizzos had found some professional success in the South, they still endured the systemic laws that framed black Americans as second-class citizens: Sit in the back of the bus out of the view of any white passengers. Pick up your food from the back of the restaurant so that the white customers don't have to be near you. Submit to white people. Never forget that they are your superiors.

African Americans endured this horrid environment for decades in order to survive. But when they could, they sought a way out. When the family moved north in 1956, they joined about six million African Americans who had left the South in hopes of a better life as a part of the Great Migration. The move proved beneficial for their daughter, Risa. She didn't experience much overt racism growing up.

Due to Risa's early exposure to medicine, she was certain that she wanted to become a physician by the time she was in ninth grade. She asked her dad if she could shadow him during one of his surgeries. Nowadays, it's not permissible for a surgeon to bring a fifteen-year-old along with them for a case. But Risa was lucky enough to gain that exposure. During my 2021 interview with Dr. Risa Lavizzo-Mourey, she recalled this distinct experience. She had entered the operating room and positioned herself next to the anesthesiologist, giving her a clear line of view to the operation. Her dad was discussing the clinical case as he took a scalpel to the skin of the patient, a young man. Risa couldn't take her eyes off of that glinting knife. Her father pressed the blade against the patient's skin and pulled back. Slowly, the wound grew bigger and bigger. Risa's widening eyes seemed to follow in sync. Whack! Her body crashed to the ground.

Everyone's attention was immediately diverted to Risa. She had passed out. The anesthesiologist rushed to remove her from the operating theater. A member of the medical team watched over Risa while everyone else continued the surgery. When Risa finally regained consciousness and realized what had happened, her face became red hot. She was so embarrassed. Her heart sunk as she assumed that she was never going to be a doctor. It just wasn't meant to be. When she relayed these feelings to her dad, he protested: "No! No! A lot of people faint the first time they go in the operating room. It's no big deal." With time, her unease about the situation slowly slipped away. Risa described the memory of her father nurturing her after this incident as "the biggest antidote to the negative things that I would hear . . . in that time, in college, and later in medical school." She learned at an early age, "you can go to ground in the operating room and still get up and be a physician."[3] If your will is strong enough, there's nothing that can hold you back.

A few years later, Risa's dad started having his own obstacles in medicine. Maybe it began with a slight stiffness when he unscrewed a bottle of jam. Or the sensation of being tipsy when he hadn't sipped a drink. But when it became challenging to tie a knot, he knew something was terribly wrong. He went to his doctor to investigate the movement challenges that he was having. To his great dismay, they delivered the diagnosis he was dreading: Parkinson's disease. Parkinson's disease is a neurodegenerative disease that depletes dopamine, a neurochemical messenger that regulates movement and mood, and aids in learning and memory. Common symptoms associated with Parkinson's disease include trembling hands and arms, stiff limbs, slowed movement, and impaired balance and coordination. This diagnosis meant the end of Dr. Philip Lavizzo's surgical career.

When Dr. Lavizzo realized this, he was utterly devastated. His love for surgery was rivaled only by his love for his family. He began taking levodopa (L-dopa), a precursor molecule to dopamine, in an attempt to slow the progression of the disease. When he fell ill, this treatment was still in the early stages of clinical use. It is now known that this drug can cause depression, likely due to the reduced levels of intrinsic dopamine in the early stages of treatment. This is followed by a rebound in mood around the same time that movement begins to improve. After decades of using this drug for Parkinson's disease patients, clinicians are now better equipped to manage that early dip in mood. Risa's dad began taking the medication only about ten years into its widespread use. He didn't have that luxury of clinical insight.

When Risa graduated from high school, the family was overjoyed. Risa had done so well that she gained a spot in Yale University's entering class of 1972. But this joy was ripped from the family when Dr. Philip

Lavizzo lost his life to suicide about a week after Risa's high school graduation. While the family knew that Dr. Lavizzo was heartbroken when he gave up his work, they never imagined that this sorrow in combination with the L-dopa treatment could have such dire consequences.

Risa was devastated. And she couldn't stop thinking about how this catastrophe was crushing her mother and her younger siblings. Overnight, Risa's mom became a grieving widow, the primary breadwinner of the household, and the sole parent of four children (including two who were under ten). It was too much. The family continued to struggle midway through the summer. So Risa deferred her matriculation to Yale by a year. She instead started college locally at the University of Washington so that she could be there for her family. This decision changed everything.

Due to the timing of the decision, Risa matriculated at the University of Washington after many of her classmates had. She was still able to enroll in some premed classes, but she had few options for her electives. Risa chose Public Health 101 as one of her electives. It was a topic she wasn't familiar with. The course provided Risa with a broad perspective on the public health initiatives that really made an impact in the community. It also made her realize that while individual medical therapies were essential to the advancement of medicine, public health was necessary to heal populations. To comprehend population health, her public health professor created a framework for social determinants of health. This concept appeared repeatedly throughout Dr. Risa Lavizzo-Mourey's career and helped her understand why many of her black patients had worse health outcomes than her white patients did.

While Risa was starting to form an idea of how she wanted her career to look, she also had to fulfill the requirements of a premedical student. One such responsibility was attending early morning science labs. She had to start her day while campus was still quiet. She made sure to give herself enough time to eat food from the student union's cafeteria before these multi-hour labs. When she arrived, she found a few students scattered throughout the dining hall. Risa gravitated toward one in particular: Robert (Bob) Mourey, a handsome young man who was in his senior year. He was also an early riser, so their breakfast meetups became a regular occurrence. As Risa got to know him, she felt a spark. There was something special about this man.

As their relationship developed, Risa made it clear that she was going to become a physician. Like Dr. Claudia Thomas, Risa had dated other guys who detested her ambition. Thankfully, Bob was different. He shared a vision of a two-career family. This, in addition to many other factors, made Risa confident that he was the one. Bob was her soul mate. So, toward the end of the school year, they promised to spend their lives together. Their engagement diverted Risa's plan to start school at Yale for her sophomore year. Instead, she moved to New York with her soon-to-be husband. They attended the State University of New York at Stony Brook together. Risa was a premedical student, and Bob was a sociology graduate student. While Risa made this early sacrifice, Bob maintained his vow to support Risa's career. The couple's decision to relocate to New York came with a promise: since Bob had chosen this move, the next choice was Risa's. They would alternate like this for the next fifty years.

Unfortunately, Risa was not happy at Stony Brook. It was a commuter school with only a handful of black students. In each of her premed classes, she was the sole melanated person in a sea full of whiteness. The only time she had other black people in her class was in the one African American history class that was offered at the school. The national trend of universities excluding the role of African Americans from much of the American history they taught negatively impacted many black students, including Risa and Claudia. Risa felt isolated at this school due to its lack of diversity, and the feeling was exacerbated by the white students' views of their black classmates.

The white students' prejudice was heighted by President John F. Kennedy's attempt to reduce the racial discrimination that permeated the country. On March 6, 1961, President Kennedy issued Executive Order 10925, which demanded that employers terminate discriminatory employment practices that were based on potential employees' ethnicity and/or nationality. The impact of affirmative action expanded beyond Kennedy's initial mandate thanks to the civil rights movement and eventual passage of civil rights legislation later in the 1960s. Affirmative action has helped white women advance in their careers more so than any other demographic, but this fact is oftentimes forgotten. Instead, people tend to focus their attention on black Americans. They claim that legislation that was meant to combat over a century of discriminatory practices instead serves to give underrepresented people advantages that they don't deserve.

This white supremacist mentality hit home for Risa in the early 1970s, when she took a course on improving health in underserved communities that was taught by well-known journalist and social activist Jack Geiger. During one class session, the topic of affirmative action came up. Instinctively, one student blurted out, "There are black people that are getting into medical school and taking seats away from more deserving white students."[4] Immediately, all heads turned to Risa. She was the only black student in that class. Despite the clear disproportionality in representation, many were convinced that she had gained access to a space that she didn't deserve to be in. They didn't realize that she had actually passed up her Yale acceptance to study at Stony Brook.

The academic excellence that gained Risa acceptance into that prestigious university continued to shine through at Stony Brook. The premed office ranked all of the students applying to medical school according to their test scores and GPAs. The ranking was posted on a counselor's door. To maintain some level of anonymity, the office used the students' Social Security numbers instead of their names. While white students were suggesting that Risa didn't earn her spot at the school, she was the highest-ranked premedical student in the entire class. No one stopped to consider how well Risa grasped the class material. And the thought that she could be performing better than every white student was surely unfathomable to them. Some people's prejudice is explicit. Others' is implicit. But the assumption is always the same: black people can't be intellectual equals to their white peers, and there's no way they can be more intelligent. It just goes against common (white) sense.

Risa was hurt by her classmates' responses, but she didn't let this deter her. She continued working hard in school. By her third year of college, in 1974, she was ready to escape the prejudiced culture at Stony Brook. She spoke to her premed counselors about applying to medical school in her third year, but they discouraged her. She had completed, and excelled in, all the prerequisite classes for medical school. But the premed counselors didn't believe that she was medical school material. It didn't matter that she had extensive experience in the hospital, dating back to her childhood, or that she was the top student in her class. In their minds, Risa's identity as a black woman disqualified her as someone who could succeed in medical school. They actually believed that applying to medical school would be a waste of her money, in spite of the ranking posted on the door.[5]

In the 1860s, Dr. Rebecca Crumpler was told that the MD at the end of her name stood for mule driver, because she surely couldn't have earned a medical degree. In the 1930s, Dr. Lena Edwards was refused acceptance into residency programs for eight consecutive years because the admissions committee believed that her identity as a black woman meant that she was incapable of becoming a competent physician. And in the 1950s, Dr. Marilyn Gaston's high school counselors tried to dissuade her from pursuing medicine because they believed her identity as a poor black girl deemed her unfit. So it's no surprise that in the 1970s, Risa's college counselors were convinced that she wouldn't succeed in medical school.

Even in 2021, the tradition lives on. I, along with countless other black medical students, have been told that we "stole a medical school spot from a more deserving nonblack medical applicant," that we "will bring down the class averages," and that we "just aren't as hardworking as our peers." At some point, these people will have to accept the truth— we can excel in this space. The proof is in our legacy of black women physicians who achieved so much in their careers, despite all the work put into keeping them out of this profession.

Risa combated this discriminatory behavior the way many of her predecessors had: by ignoring the hate and staying focused on the goal. She sent applications to ten medical schools, including all of the Ivy League medical schools, the University of Washington, and Stanford University, despite the Stony Brook advisors. Her stellar record earned her interviews from all ten of these schools. When she interviewed at Harvard Medical School, she met Deborah Meyers, an African American woman in her second year of medical school. Risa remembered looking up to her because Deborah had already survived the first year of medical school. During the interview, Risa described her career interests to Deborah. She said she felt drawn to research and thought that she would enjoy a career in academic medicine. But Risa admitted that she felt somewhat guilty pursuing this interest because she knew that African Americans needed more primary care physicians. Deborah leaned into Risa and said, "We need 'em all, honey! Whatever you want to do. We need it all."[6] Risa felt a rush of relief flood over her. With these few words, this peer-mentor gave Risa permission to just pursue her passions. She felt accepted and seen. It was something she hadn't felt since she lived with her family in Seattle. Immediately she knew that Harvard Medical School was the place she was meant to be.

After Risa completed all her interviews, there was a period of silence. Months went by without a word from the schools. She had a general idea of when she was supposed to hear back, but she didn't know the exact dates. By springtime, the admissions letters started to roll in. Yale. Columbia. University of Washington. She was so excited about these acceptances, but there was still one school she was holding her breath for.

When she received the envelope from Harvard, her heart began to race. She inspected the size of the envelope. It was thick! Ecstasy jolted through her veins. She knew that a thick envelope was good news, because it could hold the admissions decision as well as other important forms. If it was going to be a rejection, it would've been thin. So she savored the moment. She slowly separated the binding, careful not to rip the paper. Once she finally opened the envelope, she read the letter on top: an acceptance. She had been dreaming about this moment since she was a child. Her hard work finally paid off.

Now that she had been accepted into medical school, she could leave Stony Brook, even though she hadn't completed all its requirements for an undergraduate degree. At the time, medical schools required certain premed classes, but not a bachelor's degree, to matriculate. But students could typically work with their undergraduate university to attain their degree even if they left early for medical school. Risa hoped to make this arrangement with Stony Brook. She told her premed advisor about her acceptance to Harvard, along with the eight other prestigious medical schools. But they still weren't convinced that she could become a doctor. The counselor thought Risa might not make it through the training process, and they weren't shy about their doubts. They told her that she could send them her medical school transcript from the first year *if* she could make it that far.[7] They said they would give her a bachelor's degree from Stony Brook only if she submitted this medical school transcript. Risa was sick and tired of the school's lack of support. So she decided not to complete the process. She was going to earn her medical degree. She could do without the bachelor's.

In the summer of 1975, Risa and Bob got married and moved to Boston. The move thrust them into a sea of racial tensions that had been mounting for over a decade. Racism has held a strong grip on Boston throughout its history.[8] In 1861, Dr. Rebecca Crumpler literally fled Boston and moved *south* to Richmond, Virginia, because it wasn't safe for African Americans to live in Boston. A mob of white men had taken clubs, stones, and axes to beat African Americans in their North Beacon Hill neighborhood, only two miles from Dr. Crumpler's medical school, because the white people were enraged by the possibility that slavery would be outlawed in the South—and large groups of police officers just stood by and watched the violence unfold. Rebecca didn't feel safe to return to Boston and continue her medical education for two years, until the Civil War had progressed and President Abraham Lincoln had signed the Emancipation Proclamation.

While Boston was forced to adhere to early abolition legislation in Massachusetts, the city skirted the national mandate to end racial segregation under the Civil Rights Act of 1964. It maintained segregation in its public schools, prompting black Americans to engage in nonviolent protests. In 1972, after about a decade of protests, the US District Court for the District of Massachusetts finally investigated the actions of Boston public schools. In 1974, following a lengthy trial, Judge W. Arthur Garrity Jr. found that the Boston School Committee had "knowingly carried out a systematic program of segregation affecting all of the city's students, teachers, and school facilities."[9] The public schools were forced to desegregate.

White Bostonians in the 1970s mirrored the actions of white locals from more than a century before, meeting this court ruling—which increased equality—with violence. In order to desegregate the schools, Judge Garrity ordered school buses to take African American students to predominantly white schools and white students to black schools. On the opening day of classes, when this order was implemented, white adults hurled bricks and bottles at African American children who were taking the bus to school.[10] This act of violence against children spiked racial tensions in the city.

Amid the tensions, Risa and Bob tried to focus on getting settled before Risa started medical school. But whenever the couple expressed interest in an apartment that was listed as open, the landlords claimed that the units were already rented. Eventually it became clear that these units were still available, but the landlords were trying to prevent black people from moving into that area. This was the first time Risa was overtly denied something because of her race. Seattle had effectively shielded her from this harsh form of racism.

The city did not welcome Risa, but the black community at Harvard Medical School (HMS) did. She found it so refreshing to enter a space with other black people who shared her passion for medicine, especially after the challenges she faced at Stony Brook. Her black classmates were able to relate to her challenges moving to Boston. They didn't experience racism just in the medical space. Discrimination crowded them on all sides. The black medical community was a space for them to all heal from their hurtful experiences while supporting one another along their professional journeys. Dr. Alvin Poussaint was the glue for the community. He became the faculty associate dean for student affairs at HMS in 1969 and remained in that position for fifty years.[11] Over the course of his tenure, he recruited and mentored almost 1,400 students of color at the medical school.[12] He also played a central role in the formation of diversity and inclusion at HMS. The community served as Risa's lifeline as she traversed the challenges of attending HMS and living in Boston as a black woman.

This support system was essential when a white male professor at HMS published an article about affirmative action in the *New England*

Journal of Medicine. The professor thought it was wrong that it benefited black students; he wasn't as concerned about how it gave increased access to white female students. He wrote boldly that there were minority students admitted to medical school who weren't competent and were going to "leave a swath of death in their path."[13] He was one member of a larger faction of professors who, even within the ivied walls of their own medical school, tried to snatch any confidence black students had in their ability to succeed in medicine.

Racist incidents like this were surely painful, but like Drs. Edith Irby Jones and Marilyn Gaston, Risa refused to let prejudiced people impede her progress toward her goals. She hunkered down and tried to keep her focus fixed on the demands of a rigorous medical school curriculum. As she progressed through her training, she found herself increasingly drawn to internal medicine. She believed that she could study the topics that she found intellectually challenging, such as the social determinants of health, from the perch of internal medicine. After Dr. Risa Lavizzo-Mourey graduated from HMS in 1979, she started an internal medicine residency at Brigham and Women's Hospital, an affiliate of the medical school.

During Dr. Lavizzo-Mourey's residency training, she felt that she was ready to make progress in another area of her life: having a baby. She had her first child, her daughter, during residency; she had her son right before starting her fellowship. This timing worked out well because her postgraduate training had clear demarcations between work and personal life. During work hours, she was expected to be present. But when she left the hospital and wasn't on call, her time was her own. There was an expectation to read medical journals to expand her knowledge and be a good doctor, but this reading could be done on her schedule. In contrast, once she became an attending physician and assistant professor, it was as if she were working 24/7. She had to teach and be on call for her patients, as well as write grants and fulfill other administrative duties. Her husband's support with the family's needs made the balance between Dr. Lavizzo-Mourey's family and career responsibilities more manageable.

Once Dr. Lavizzo-Mourey completed her residency, it was her husband's turn to choose where the family moved. He chose Philadelphia.

Dr. Lavizzo-Mourey had previously secured a fellowship in hypertension with Dr. Victor Dzau when he was working at Brigham and Women's Hospital. (Dzau is currently the president of the United States National Academy of Medicine, having served in this position since 2014. Before this, he served as president and CEO of Duke University Medical Center.) Because Risa and her husband were on different career timelines, she had to apply for fellowships before her husband knew where he would be hired. So when he landed his sociology teaching job in Philly, Dr. Lavizzo-Mourey was put in a difficult position. She was excited about the fellowship opportunity with Dr. Dzau, but she had made a promise to her husband. Managing a dual-career household did not come without its hitches, but this family was committed to making it work.

Dr. Lavizzo-Mourey didn't want a long commute to work, so she gave up an incredible fellowship opportunity and began interviewing for jobs in Philly. She landed a job as a primary care physician with a new practice that Temple University had opened in Center City, Philadelphia. After working in this position for two years, Dr. Lavizzo-Mourey realized that she didn't want to work in traditional primary care. Most of her patients were young and healthy. The experience contrasted with her time in medical training, when she had cared for really sick patients. One patient population that she did enjoy in Philly was the geriatric patient population. Their clinical presentations were intellectually challenging, and caring for them was emotionally rewarding. Because they were often ignored, she knew she was making a difference by giving them the care that they deserved. A clinical practice in geriatrics also aligned with her research interests in health policy in the context of Medicare.

Dr. Lavizzo-Mourey left Temple and joined the Robert Wood Johnson Foundation (RWJF) Clinical Scholars fellowship program, which was affiliated with the University of Pennsylvania. Dr. Lavizzo-Mourey was still interested in exploring population-based healthcare, but Penn didn't have a school of public health at the time. So, she crafted her own program to explore her varied interests. She simultaneously worked on her RWJF fellowship and an MBA in healthcare administration at the

Wharton School of the University of Pennsylvania. In 1986, Dr. Lavizzo-Mourey completed the fellowship in general internal medicine with a focus in geriatrics and the MBA. She did all this as a new mom who had given birth to her second child about six weeks before starting the fellowship. Once she completed her training, she became an assistant professor at the Perelman School of Medicine and at Wharton. Six years later, in 1992, she was promoted to associate professor at the Perelman School of Medicine and at Wharton.

Dr. Lavizzo-Mourey was very successful in academic medicine, but entering this space did pose some challenges. Throughout her medical training, she had had a community of other black physicians whom she could relate to. Once she reached faculty level, it was just her and one other African American. She no longer had that community of medical colleagues who could both share recipes for cherished soul food dishes and understand the pain of yet another nonblack colleague mistaking them for a nurse's aide instead of an attending physician. This academic environment also demanded collaborative research. But because there were few black physicians on the faculty, Dr. Lavizzo-Mourey faced challenges finding colleagues who also wanted to study the health disparities impacting the African American population.

Dr. Lavizzo-Mourey found her early faculty years particularly difficult due to this stark shift in her environment. It made her feel isolated and out of place. Countless black physicians have reported similar feelings of isolation within academic medicine.[14] This is one of many issues that contribute to the underrepresentation of black physicians in academia. Less than 2 percent of physicians in academic medicine are black women, and only 0.7 percent of medical school faculty full professors are black women.[15] While Dr. Risa Lavizzo-Mourey experienced many challenges within academic medicine, she drew strength from the community of black physicians whom she knew outside of her institution. Leveraging a community of black professionals to cope is a popular strategy used by black physicians in this position. Dr. May Chinn found community through friends who were also leaders of the Harlem Renaissance. Dr. Dorothy Ferebee found her community through Alpha Kappa Alpha Sorority and other black professional organizations.

Having this community reminds people that they're not alone in their struggles, which makes it easier for them to navigate obstacles.

One way that Dr. Lavizzo-Mourey cultivated her community of black professionals was by attending annual conferences hosted by the Association of Academic Minority Physicians (AAMP). This organization had been founded in 1986 by six black male academic physicians who held prominent and visible positions in academia, including Dr. Louis W. Sullivan and Dr. Donald E. Wilson. At the time of the organization's founding, these physicians recognized that underrepresented minorities "accounted for only 3% of U.S. medical school faculty, 1.9% of professors, and no academic Dean . . . (except for traditionally minority schools)."[16] These six physicians wanted to create an organization that would diversify medicine and, as a result, improve health outcomes in the US for minority populations. One strategy that they used to work toward these goals was to foster a community among physicians in academia.

Three years after helping to create the AAMP, Dr. Sullivan was appointed secretary of the US Department of Health and Human Services by President George H. W. Bush. Before holding this position, Dr. Sullivan had been founding dean and president of the Morehouse School of Medicine. Dr. Sullivan worked for the White House throughout the elder Bush's presidency, from 1989 to 1993. One of Dr. Sullivan's key initiatives during his tenure was to increase gender and ethnic diversity in senior positions at the Department of Health and Human Services. He helped to appoint the first (white) female director of the National Institutes of Health, and the first female and first Latinx surgeon general of the United States. In addition to his role in making these high-profile appointments, Dr. Sullivan enlisted the help of a few of his long-term colleagues to help him identify other minority physicians who could make a positive impact in the department.

Dr. Donald E. Wilson was one of Dr. Sullivan's trusted advisors. In 1991, Dr. Wilson became the country's first African American dean of a medical school that was not historically black when he joined the University of Maryland School of Medicine. That same year, he made a call to Dr. Lavizzo-Mourey. Dr. Wilson wanted to gauge Dr. Lavizzo-Mourey's interest in going to Washington, DC, to join Dr. Sullivan's Agency for

Health Care Policy and Research. This government job was a great op-portunity for Dr. Lavizzo-Mourey to explore her public health interests, but she felt hampered by the circumstances of the offer. First, she was a lifelong Democrat, and this was a Republican administration. She wasn't sure she would fit in. Second, she had another year or so before she would go up for tenure. Without that job security, taking a leave of absence to pursue this policy job could threaten her position at Penn. Election to the tenure track relied on standardized guidelines, such as publishing a certain number of papers in academic journals. While she was making promising strides toward this benchmark, a hiatus could stall her. Lastly, she would have to commute from Philly to Maryland to work, but she had two young children. She wanted to be as present with her kids as possible.

All of these factors made her hesitant to accept the position. Her advisors discouraged her from taking the job. But she had a nagging voice that kept saying, "You've always said that you want to work on expanding access to coverage. Here's a chance to do it."[17] While ramp-ing up support for his second presidential race, Bush had been saying that he wanted to increase the number of beneficiaries of Medicare. Dr. Lavizzo-Mourey wanted to be a part of this expansion. In 1992, she took a calculated risk and accepted the job.

Dr. Lavizzo-Mourey was considered for a presidential appointment by the Bush administration, but officials quickly found out that she wasn't a Republican. As a result, she was brought on the team under the senior executive service, the civil service, instead of via presidential appointment. When President Bush lost the election to Bill Clinton and his administration ended, all the presidential appointees were expected to resign. Since Dr. Lavizzo-Mourey was a member of the civil service, she kept her job. She remained vocal about her interest in healthcare reform, so President Clinton appointed her to serve as cochair of the quality of care working group of the White House Task Force on Health Care Reform. Although the three doctors may not have overlapped, there was a brief period when Drs. Marilyn Gaston, Joycelyn Elders, and Risa Lavizzo-Mourey were all working at the White House to address various public health concerns.

Dr. Lavizzo-Mourey's experience working on the presidential committees taught her the inner workings of the highest levels of government; she saw how difficult it was to bring a significant piece of legislation to Congress and then get it passed. It required a team to produce extensive research, work with Congress, and bring vital constituencies on board. There were many limitations to the process. While the Clinton administration tried its best, it failed to expand healthcare coverage. Through this journey, Dr. Lavizzo-Mourey became a leader in healthcare reform and in battling health disparities impacting African American and Latinx communities. Whenever someone wanted to make an impact in this space, they called Dr. Lavizzo-Mourey. Those two years gave her a more focused perspective on how to make a greater impact.

There was a maximum amount of time that Penn allotted for faculty to take leave to work in high-level government agency positions while maintaining their faculty positions. As Dr. Lavizzo-Mourey neared that time limit, she had to decide if she would stay in government or go back to academia. Throughout her time working for the government, she had had to commute. She would leave Philly on a Sunday night and come back Friday afternoon. Her family was proud of the impact Dr. Lavizzo-Mourey was making in society, but they still missed her at home. One Sunday night when she was putting her son to bed, he said, "You know, we've been living in different cities for two years. Don't you think it's time we all lived in the same place?"

Her son's plea struck her heart. Risa thought to herself, "This is not good. I need to come on home."[18]

So, in 1994, she rejoined the faculty at Penn, where she was given a lot more responsibility. Suddenly, the senior faculty viewed her as someone who could actually run things, as someone who understood policy making. Within the year, she was promoted to chief of the division of geriatric medicine, director at the Institute on Aging, associate dean for health services research, and associate executive vice president for health policy, all at the University of Pennsylvania. In 1995, she was also appointed Sylvan Eisman Professor of Medicine at the Perelman School of Medicine. After working in these roles for more than five years, she started thinking about her next steps.

She received multiple offers for higher-level positions within academia, but she wasn't sure if they were the right move for her. Academia's focus was feeling more and more constraining for what she wanted to do. She wanted to make change on a broader level. She was offered a job as senior vice president at the Robert Wood Johnson Foundation. This offer piqued her interest because she was familiar with the impact RWJF had on healthcare. She also knew that the foundation would be appointing a new president soon. She believed that her unique passions and skills made her ideally suited to lead the organization.

Then she considered the organization's long history of white male presidents. "In my mind, I didn't think it was such a long shot. Although almost everyone else thought it was a long shot. And it was. I mean, they were not thinking about a black woman for this job."[19] She knew three men working for the foundation, and many external candidates, were vying for the position. She thought it was unlikely that they interviewed any black women besides her. Diversity wasn't their focus at the time. Still, she wouldn't let that discourage her.

It was her dream job. Her experience in government made her aware of how influential foundations could be. A foundation could determine what research was needed to push forward an agenda, fund that research, and publicize it. The organization could develop a strategy and relentlessly chip away at it. Unlike a presidential administration that was limited to four or eight years, a foundation could work toward the same goal for ten years or more. It could develop a multipronged, long-term strategy that included training new health policy personnel, building community coalitions, fostering the support of political leaders, and so much more. With the time and resources that the Robert Wood Johnson Foundation could offer, Dr. Lavizzo-Mourey could tackle big problems.

In light of this offer, Penn gave her the option to take a leave of absence while holding on to her tenure. If, after a year, she wasn't appointed to president of the foundation and she wasn't happy with her job as senior vice president, she could go back to her faculty position at Penn. Even when she considered her family, there were few downsides. Her children were a bit older and more independent. Also, Princeton,

New Jersey—where her new office would be—was only about an hour's drive from Philly. The commute would be easy. This opportunity just felt right, so she accepted.

A year later, Dr. Lavizzo-Mourey received the news that she had been appointed president and CEO of the Robert Wood Johnson Foundation. She was over the moon and felt humbled by the responses. News organizations rushed to write the story; a *New York Times* article dated October 6, 2002, reported, "At age 48, a doctor specializing in geriatrics, Dr. Lavizzo-Mourey is still exploring the connection [between insurance and medical care] and—like her parents, but on a national stage—juggling the needs of health care providers and the uninsured. In December she will become the chief executive of the Robert Wood Johnson Foundation here, the nation's largest philanthropy devoted to health and health care. She will be the first woman and the first African American to head the foundation, which has an endowment of about $8 billion and distributes more than $400 million a year."[20]

Dr. Lavizzo-Mourey was honored to hold the position, but in taking it she accepted a big responsibility. Dr. Lavizzo-Mourey held the same perspective that Dr. Claudia Thomas did, a conviction echoed in Vice President Kamala Harris's first postelection address to the nation: "While I may be the first woman in this office, I will not be the last."[21] Dr. Lavizzo-Mourey wanted her presence to change the way the foundation thought about black people and women as leaders in medicine. She didn't want to just hold a seat.

As president and CEO, Dr. Lavizzo-Mourey was responsible for guiding the foundation's strategy for impact, and for working with RWJF's board of trustees and staff to implement it. Her biggest fear was that she would lead the foundation to do a lot of work and spend a lot of money but have nothing to show for it. Unsurprisingly, the opposite happened. She led the foundation to pursue five strategies that sought to change people's mindset and build a culture of health. She wanted to move the nation away from considering healthcare only in the context of the hospital, clinic, or office. Instead, she pushed people to embrace external factors—now known as social determinants of health. She believed that by addressing these factors, people would have better health outcomes and the horrid disparities in health between races and socio-economic classes of Americans would be reduced.

One such strategy the foundation employed was addressing the numerous structural factors that have contributed to the increase in childhood obesity. The foundation wanted people to stop blaming the kids' habits, or a mom's food choices, for this national crisis. Instead, the Robert Wood Johnson Foundation wanted society and policy makers to consider the societal changes that have facilitated the phenomenon. What lunch choices are offered at school? How expensive is healthy food, and how can it be made more affordable and available in food deserts? By changing the focus, the foundation might motivate people with the power to make these systemic changes to do so.

Over the course of Dr. Lavizzo-Mourey's tenure, RWJF committed a billion dollars to start a national movement to raise awareness of the childhood obesity epidemic, while also funding research, communications campaigns, and public policy advocacy. The foundation began this initiative in 2007 and planned to continue its efforts for at least two decades. It collaborated with schools, industry, policy makers, cities, and organizations to work toward its ambitious goal of making healthy food and activities, like sports, accessible to children across the nation. These dynamic efforts even attracted high-profile leaders, such as First Lady Michelle Obama, who decided to adopt the foundation's focus on childhood obesity through her "Let's Move!" campaign.[22]

The success of this initiative is evident in the national trends. The Centers for Disease Control and Prevention reported a staggering increase in obesity, from 5 percent to 17 percent, among children aged two to nineteen between 1976 and 2007.[23] But in the nine years since the RWJF began this initiative, obesity rates have held steady at 17 percent.[24] Even more remarkable, the rate of obesity among preschool age children (two to five years) decreased significantly, from 13.9 percent to 8.4 percent from 2003 to 2014.[25] Dr. Lavizzo-Mourey led the RWJF in one of its boldest health initiatives, which will have a long-lasting impact on the health of Americans around the country.

Still, she believed that the foundation could do more. Under her direction, the RWJF in 2008 established the Commission to Build a

Healthier America, a national independent, nonpartisan coalition of leaders working to identify the factors outside of medical care that impact health. After spending a year collecting data and speaking to Americans across the country, the commission reported its findings in "Beyond Health Care."[26] The report stressed the importance of social determinants of health—the idea that where people live, learn, work, and play can have a bigger impact on their health than medical care itself.

Based on this insight, the commission provided national recommendations aimed at improving health at the local, state, and federal levels. It advocated for collaboration between the public and private sectors, and for continuity of funding so that initiatives could be fully implemented. The efforts aimed to remove barriers to health, for example, by providing transportation for people who struggle to access healthcare and pharmacies, while creating opportunities to promote more healthful behaviors, such as by preserving green spaces in urban areas to encourage more active lifestyles while improving mental health. The commission identified income and education levels as the two most critical, yet most challenging, factors that needed to be addressed before health disparities could truly be reduced and sustained improvements in health outcomes for all Americans were seen. The commission's findings led Dr. Lavizzo-Mourey, with the full backing of the RWJF board, to create programming inspired by the foundation's current vision for building a culture of health in America—reducing health disparities by addressing the social determinants of health as outlined by the commission. The effort is a multilayered, long-term initiative, similar to the childhood obesity initiative.

Dr. Lavizzo-Mourey's impact on American society is one that cannot be fully measured. In a 2016 interview, the RWJF board of trustees chairman, Roger Fine, explained: "Risa's commitment to improving the health of this nation during her tenure as CEO is simply unparalleled, and she has led this Foundation with an extraordinary sense of purpose and passion."[27] Dr. Lavizzo-Mourey's impact has been recognized by numerous organizations, including *Forbes*, which has named her one of the world's most powerful women eight times, and *Modern Healthcare*, which has named her one of the hundred most influential people in healthcare nine times.

Like the other black women physicians in this book, Dr. Risa Lavizzo-Mourey faced off against a system designed for black women to fail, and not only did she succeed by becoming a great physician; she used her privileged position to make medicine more accessible for those coming after her, while working tirelessly to improve the health of a sector of Americans who are too often overlooked. When she gave me advice on how I could make an impact in medicine while developing other important areas of my life, she eloquently explained, "You're going to have to make sacrifices to do something bigger than yourself. That's always the case. But you've also got to make sure that you take care of all of those parts of your life and weave it all together."[28]

REMEMBER THEIR STORIES

It was mid-August 2021. The sweltering Philadelphia heat tried to dampen my mood, but I was too excited for my first day back to medical school. I'd spent a long year watching virtual lectures alone in my apartment, and we were finally having class in person! I craved the camaraderie that came from tackling this difficult material shoulder-to-shoulder with the rest of my class. It would make the grueling process much more enjoyable.

As I tried to locate the room for my first cardiology lecture, I felt lost. The long halls with marble-accented walls seemed to blend into each other. Initially, I felt like I was going in circles, but eventually I started to make headway. As I neared my lecture hall, I became engulfed in a row of portraits depicting old white men, their eyes looking down on me. A brief glance at the labels below their ornate frames revealed that these were all physicians and/or scientists; these were the people my school believed were important to memorialize. Despite perusing dozens of portraits, I couldn't find a single woman or black person portrayed on the walls. This hall reminded me of the history lessons I was taught from elementary school through to my master's degree in history of medicine. Almost every physician that my schools taught me about were white men; none of them were black women.

A few years ago, this hall would've bothered me. Like my history lessons, it conveyed the message that I, as a black woman, will not be able to make a significant contribution to the medical field. My identities preclude me from being able to have an impact worth remembering.

The words of prejudiced peers and leaders in society reinforce this idea. As a black person I don't have the intellectual capabilities to succeed in medicine. As a woman I don't have the innate skills to be a leader. While I didn't believe this bigoted perspective, I used to wonder if people's bias would hinder my advancement in my career.

But as I embarked on this journey to uncover the stories of black women physicians, I learned a new truth. Black women have been leaders in medicine in America for over 150 years, despite the immense barriers erected along their paths. They've succeeded in medical specialties, surgical specialties, public health, and policy while providing care for underserved communities on the local, national, and international levels. They've changed the culture of medicine, making the field more accessible for women and people of color coming behind them. And they've shone a light on structural problems within medicine that have led to subpar care in black and brown communities while they worked to change the system from within.

When I look at the portraits of these old white men and note the absence of portraits commemorating physicians who look like me, I feel at peace. The triumph of black women physicians has etched itself into my memory. Their victories shape the way I walk in medical spaces, and serve as a shield against the physicians, medical students, and patients who have questioned my ability to become a competent physician. I now know that I, a black woman, can have an immense impact in medicine. I may have to work twice as hard as my colleagues with more privileged identities, but eventually I will become a changemaker within medicine, positively impacting patients and aspiring physicians within my reach.

NOTES

PROLOGUE

1. Ellen Craft Dammond, "Black Women Oral History Project. Interviews, 1976–1981. May Edward Chinn," *Harvard Library Viewer*, Schlesinger Library, Radcliffe College (December 11, 1981): 23.
2. Tom W. Smith, "Changing Racial Labels: From 'Colored' to 'Negro' to 'Black' to 'African American,'" *Public Opinion Quarterly* 56 (1992): 499.
3. Smith, "Changing Racial Labels," 503.
4. Association of American Medical Colleges, "Diversity in Medical Education: Facts & Figures 2016—Current Trends in Medical Education," figure 6, https://www .aamcdiversityfactsandfigures2016.org/report-section/section-3/#figure-6.

CHAPTER 1: WITH DETERMINATION AND FEARLESSNESS

1. E. Richard Brown, *Rockefeller Medicine Men: Medicine and Capitalism in America* (Berkeley: University of California Press, 1981), 61.
2. Howard Markel, "Celebrating Rebecca Lee Crumpler, First African-American Woman Physician," *PBS NewsHour*, last modified March 9, 2016, https://www.pbs .org/newshour/health/celebrating-rebecca-lee-crumpler-first-african-american -physician.
3. "Women in the University," University of Glasgow, https://www.universitystory .gla.ac.uk/women-background, accessed April 9, 2022.
4. John Stauffer, *The Works of James McCune Smith: Black Intellectual and Abolitionist* (New York: Oxford University Press, 1964), xxi.
5. Bryan Greene, "America's First Black Physician Sought to Heal a Nation's Persistent Illness," *Smithsonian*, February 2021, https://www.smithsonianmag.com/history /james-mccune-smith-america-first-black-physician-180977110.
6. Bill O'Driscoll, "Free at Last? Tells How Slavery in Pennsylvania Ended: Slowly," *Pittsburgh City Paper*, March 26, 2009, https://www.pghcitypaper.com/pittsburgh /free-at-last-tells-how-slavery-in-pennsylvania-ended-slowly/Content?oid=1341692.
7. Marc J. Kahn and Ernest J. Sneed, "Promoting the Affordability of Medical Education to Groups Underrepresented in the Profession: The Other Side of the Equation," *AMA Journal of Ethics* 17, no. 2 (February 2015): 172–75.
8. Peggy Chambers, *A Doctor Alone: A Biography of Elizabeth Blackwell, the First Woman Doctor, 1821–1910* (London: Bodley Head, 1956).
9. Chambers, *A Doctor Alone.*
10. Laura Clark, "The First Woman in America to Receive an M.D. Was Admitted to Med School as a Joke," *Smithsonian*, January 2015, https://www.smithsonian

mag.com/smart-news/first-woman-america-receive-md-was-admitted-med
-school-joke-180953978.

11. Chambers, *A Doctor Alone.*

12. Jaclyn Long, "Rebecca Lee Crumpler: Physician, Author, Pioneer," *SITNBoston*
(blog), Harvard Graduate School of Arts and Sciences, last modified December 24,
2020, https://sitn.hms.harvard.edu/flash/2020/rebecca-lee-crumpler-physician
-author-pioneer.

13. Markel, "Celebrating Rebecca Lee Crumpler, First African-American Woman
Physician."

14. "The Gathering Storm: The Secession Crisis," American Battlefield Trust, https://
www.battlefields.org/learn/articles/gathering-storm-secession-crisis, accessed
March 1, 2022.

15. Patrick T. J. Browne, "'This Most Atrocious Crusade Against Personal Freedom':
Anti-Abolitionist Violence in Boston on the Eve of War," *New England Quarterly*
94, no. 1 (2021): 47–81.

16. "The John Brown Anniversary Meeting," Museum of African American History,
https://www.smithcourtstories.org/the-john-brown-anniversary-meeting, accessed
April 8, 2022.

17. "Acknowledging Dr. Rebecca Crumpler," Resilient Sisterhood Project, last modified June 22, 2021, https://www.rsphealth.org/dr-rebecca-crumpler.

18. "Acknowledging Dr. Rebecca Crumpler."

19. "Acknowledging Dr. Rebecca Crumpler."

20. "Freedmen's Bureau Acts of 1865 and 1866," Art & History, US Senate, https://
www.senate.gov/artandhistory/history/common/generic/FreedmensBureau.htm,
accessed March 1, 2022.

21. Long, "Rebecca Lee Crumpler: Physician, Author, Pioneer."

22. Sarah K. A. Pfatteicher, "Rebecca Davis Lee Crumpler," in *African American Lives*,
ed. Henry Louis Gates Jr. and Evelyn Brooks Higginbotham (New York: Oxford
University Press, 2004), 199–200.

23. "Dr. Rebecca Lee Crumpler," Changing the Face of Medicine, National Library
of Medicine, National Institutes of Health, last modified June 3, 2015, https://cf
medicine.nlm.nih.gov/physicians/biography_73.html.

24. Long, "Rebecca Lee Crumpler: Physician, Author, Pioneer."

25. Myron Schultz, "Rudolf Virchow," *Emerging Infectious Diseases* 14, no. 9 (2008):
1480–81; Steven A. Edwards, "Rudolph Virchow, the Father of Cellular Pathology,"
American Association for the Advancement of Science, last modified January 16,
2013, https://www.aaas.org/rudolph-virchow-father-cellular-pathology.

26. S. Nassir Ghaemi, "Biomedical Reductionist, Humanist, and Biopsychosocial
Models in Medicine," in *Handbook of the Philosophy of Medicine*, ed. T. Schramme
and S. Edwards (Dordrecht: Springer, 2015), 1–19.

27. "Louis Pasteur," Science History Institute, last modified December 14, 2017, https://
www.sciencehistory.org/historical-profile/louis-pasteur.

28. Sam Wong, "Robert Koch," *New Scientist*, https://www.newscientist.com/people
/robert-koch.

29. "Robert Koch: Biographical," Nobel Prize Foundation, https://www.nobelprize
.org/prizes/medicine/1905/koch/biographical, accessed April 11, 2022.

30. "Louis Pasteur."

31. Brown, *Rockefeller Medicine Men*, 73.
32. Brown, *Rockefeller Medicine Men*, 74.
33. Rebecca Lee Crumpler, *A Book of Medical Discourses: In Two Parts* (Boston: Cashman, Keating & Co., 1883).
34. Markel, "Celebrating Rebecca Lee Crumpler."
35. "Dr. Rebecca J. Cole," Changing the Face of Medicine, National Library of Medicine, National Institutes of Health, last modified June 3, 2015, https://cfmedicine .nlm.nih.gov/physicians/biography_66.html.

CHAPTER 2: DOING SURGERY IN THE BEDROOM

1. Patrick S. Allen, "'We Must Attack the System': The Print Practice of Black 'Doctresses,'" *Arizona Quarterly: A Journal of American Literature, Culture, and Theory* 74, no. 4 (2018): 109.
2. H. A. Callis, "The Need and Training of Negro Physicians," *Journal of Negro Education* 4, no. 1 (1936): 32–33; Ellen S. More, Elizabeth Fee, and Manon Parry, eds., *Women Physicians and the Cultures of Medicine* (Baltimore: Johns Hopkins University Press, 2009), 2.
3. United States, and US Census Bureau, *Statistical Abstract of the United States* (Washington: US GPO, 1901), No. 3—Population of the United States at Each Census, from 1790 to 1900—Continued, https://www2.census.gov/prod2/statcomp /documents/1901–02.pdf.
4. Brown, *Rockefeller Medicine Men*, 63–74.
5. Brown, *Rockefeller Medicine Men*, 64.
6. Brown, *Rockefeller Medicine Men*, 83.
7. Brown, *Rockefeller Medicine Men*, 148.
8. Brown, *Rockefeller Medicine Men*, 139–40.
9. Brown, *Rockefeller Medicine Men*, 154.
10. Brown, *Rockefeller Medicine Men*, 144.
11. Brown, *Rockefeller Medicine Men*, 148.
12. Brown, *Rockefeller Medicine Men*.
13. Earl H. Harley, "The Forgotten History of Defunct Black Medical Schools in the 19th and 20th Centuries and the Impact of the Flexner Report," *Journal of the National Medical Association* 98, no. 9 (2006), https://www.ncbi.nlm.nih.gov/pmc /articles/PMC2569729/pdf/jnma00196–0027.pdf.
14. Ann Steinecke and Charles Terrel, "Progress for Whose Future? The Impact of the Flexner Report on Medical Education for Racial and Ethnic Minority Physicians in the United States," *Academic Medicine: Journal of the Association of American Medical Colleges* 85, no. 2 (2010): 236–45, https://pubmed.ncbi.nlm.nih.gov/20107348; Lynn E. Miller and Richard M. Weiss, "Revisiting Black Medical School Extinctions in the Flexner Era," *Journal of the History of Medicine and Allied Sciences* 67, no. 2 (April 2012): 217–43, https://pubmed.ncbi.nlm.nih.gov/21296769.
15. Brown, *Rockefeller Medicine Men*, 153.
16. Allen, "We Must Attack the System," 109.
17. "Progress for African-American Pioneers in Medicine Yesterday, Today and Tomorrow," *Doctor Gator, College of Medicine News*, University of Florida College of Medicine, February 26, 2009, https://news.drgator.ufl.edu/2009/02/26/progress -for-african-american-pioneers-in-medicine-yesterday-today-and-tomorrow;

Harriet A. Washington, "Apology Shines Light on Racial Schism in Medicine," *New York Times*, July 29, 2008, https://www.nytimes.com/2008/07/29/health/views/29essa.html.

18. Christopher Klein, "Last Hired, First Fired: How the Great Depression Affected African Americans," History.com, last modified August 31, 2018, https://www.history.com/news/last-hired-first-fired-how-the-great-depression-affected-african-americans.

19. May Edward Chinn, interview by Ellen Craft Dammond, September 12, 1979, OH-31, Interviews of the Black Women Oral History Project, 1976–1981, Schlesinger Library, Radcliffe Institute, Harvard University.

20. Chinn, interview, 15.

21. Chinn, interview.

22. Chinn, interview.

23. Chinn, interview, 23.

24. Chinn, interview, 22.

25. Chinn, interview, 39.

26. Chinn, interview, 87.

27. Edward Glaeser, *Triumph of the City: How Our Greatest Invention Makes Us Richer, Smarter, Greener, Healthier, and Happier* (New York: Penguin Press, 2011), 75.

28. "2022 Best Medical Schools: Research," *U.S. News & World Report*, https://www.usnews.com/best-graduate-schools/top-medical-schools/research-rankings, accessed March 1, 2022.

29. Chinn, interview, 43.

30. Chinn, interview, 44–46.

31. "The Ku Klux Klan in the 1920s," *American Experience*, PBS, https://www.pbs.org/wgbh/americanexperience/features/flood-klan, accessed March 1, 2022.

32. Association of American Medical Colleges, "Percentage of Full-Time U.S. Medical School Faculty by Sex, Race/Ethnicity, and Rank, 2018," in *Diversity in Medicine: Facts and Figures 2019*, https://www.aamc.org/data-reports/workforce/interactive-data/figure-17-percentage-full-time-us-medical-school-faculty-sex-race/ethnicity-and-rank-2018; Christopher L. Bennett et al., "Two Decades of Little Change: An Analysis of U.S. Medical School Basic Science Faculty by Sex, Race/Ethnicity, and Academic Rank," *PLOS ONE* 15, no. 7 (2020), https://journals.plos.org/plosone/article?id=10.1371/journal.pone.0235190.

33. Chinn, interview, 56.

34. Chinn, interview.

35. Chinn, interview, 57–60.

36. Katie Goldberg, "Which Cancer Center Was First? The Answer Depends on What You Mean by 'Cancer Center,'" *Cancer Letter* 47, no. 27 (July 9, 2021), https://cancerletter.com/in-the-archives/20210709_6.

CHAPTER 3: DOING GOOD IN THE COMMUNITY

1. Stephen David Kantrowitz, *More Than Freedom: Fighting for Black Citizenship in a White Republic, 1829–1889* (New York: Penguin Random House, 2013).

2. Allen, "We Must Attack the System," 109; Richard Sandomir, "Edith Irby Jones, Barrier-Breaking Doctor in the South, Dies at 91," *New York Times*, July 23, 2019, https://www.nytimes.com/2019/07/23/obituaries/dr-edith-irby-jones-dead.html.

3. Olivia B. Waxman, "'It's a Struggle They Will Wage Alone.' How Black Women Won the Right to Vote," *Time*, last modified August 17, 2020, https://time.com /5876456/black-women-right-to-vote; "Voting Rights Act of 1965," History.com, last modified January 26, 2021, https://www.history.com/topics/black-history /voting-rights-act.

4. Dorothy Boulding Ferebee, interview by Merze Tate, January 10, 1980, OH-31, Interviews of the Black Women Oral History Project, 1976–1981, Schlesinger Library, Radcliffe Institute, Harvard University, reel 1, tape 1.

5. Ferebee, interview, reel 1, tape 1.

6. Ferebee, interview, reel 1, tape 1.

7. Ferebee, interview, reel 1, tape 1.

8. Ferebee, interview, reel 1, tape 1.

9. Ferebee, interview, reel 1, tape 1.

10. Ferebee, interview, reel 1, tape 2.

11. Ferebee, interview, reel 1, tape 4.

12. Ferebee, interview, 12.

13. Robert M. White, "Unraveling the Tuskegee Study of Untreated Syphilis," *Archives of Internal Medicine* 160, no. 5 (March 13, 2000): 585-98, https://jamanetwork.com /journals/jamainternalmedicine/fullarticle/224795.

14. "The 1938 Mississippi Health Project: Fourth Annual Report of the Alpha Kappa Alpha Sorority, December 1938," Sophia Smith Collection of Women's History, Smith College Libraries, https://libex.smith.edu/omeka/files/original/4a63a0dabde cb82dcf710a0e03979391.pdf.

15. Ferebee, interview, 28.

16. Bessie E. Cobbs, "Health on Wheels in Mississippi: The Mississippi Rural Health Project of the Alpha Kappa Alpha Sorority," *American Journal of Nursing* 41, no. 5 (May 1941): 551–54, https://www.jstor.org/stable/3415336.

17. Denise Watson, "Norfolk Native, a Pioneer in Health Care and Civil Rights, to Be Honored at Home. Finally," *Virginian-Pilot*, December 3, 2017, https://www .pilotonline.com/news/article_87bb8089–78dd-5838–84fa-14f68ae8b4ab.html.

18. Ferebee, interview, 34.

CHAPTER 4: FROM HER FAMILY FORWARD

1. Marc J. Kahn and Ernest J. Sneed, "Promoting the Affordability of Medical Education to Groups Underrepresented in the Profession: The Other Side of the Equation," *AMA Journal of Ethics* 17, no. 2 (February 2015): 172–75, https://journalofethics .ama-assn.org/sites/journalofethics.ama-assn.org/files/2018–05/oped1–1502.pdf.

2. Kahn and Sneed, "Promoting the Affordability of Medical Education to Groups Underrepresented in the Profession."

3. Brown, *Rockefeller Medicine Men*.

4. Thomas D. Snyder, "120 Years of American Education: A Statistical Portrait," National Center for Education Statistics, January 1993, 8, https://nces.ed.gov/pubs93 /93442.pdf.

5. Lena Frances Edwards-Madison, interview by Merze Tate, November 14, 1977, OH-31, Interviews of the Black Women Oral History Project, 1976–1981, Schlesinger Library, Radcliffe Institute, Harvard University, 2.

6. Edwards-Madison, interview, 3.

7. Edwards-Madison, interview, 3.
8. Reginald Oh, "Interracial Marriage in the Shadows of Jim Crow: Racial Segregation as a System of Racial and Gender Subordination," *UC Davis Law Review* 39, no. 3 (2006): 1321–52, https://lawreview.law.ucdavis.edu/issues/39/3/defining -voices-critical-race-feminism/davisvol39no3_oh.pdf.
9. Chinn, interview, 51.
10. Edwards-Madison, interview, 4.
11. "Dr. Marie Metoyer (MD '51) Leaves Lasting Legacy," Alumni News & Updates, Weill Cornell Medicine, last modified November 23, 2020, https://alumni.weill .cornell.edu/programs-events/news/dr-marie-metoyer-md-51-leaves-lasting-legacy.
12. Edwards-Madison, interview, 5.
13. "Dr. Lena Frances Edwards," Changing the Face of Medicine, National Library of Medicine, National Institutes of Health, last modified June 3, 2015, https://cf medicine.nlm.nih.gov/physicians/biography_96.html.
14. Edwards-Madison, interview, 5.
15. Edwards-Madison, interview, 5–6.
16. David R. Francis, "Employers' Replies to Racial Names," *The Digest* (National Bureau of Economic Research), no. 9 (September 2003), https://www.nber.org /digest/sep03/employers-replies-racial-names; S. Michael Gaddis, "Discrimination in the Credential Society: An Audit Study of Race and College Selectivity in the Labor Market," *Social Forces* 93, no. 4 (2015): 1451–79; and Marianne Bertrand and Sendhil Mullainathan, "Discrimination in the Job Market in the United States," Abdul Latif Jameel Poverty Action Lab, https://www.povertyactionlab.org /evaluation/discrimination-job-market-united-states, accessed March 1, 2022.
17. Edwards-Madison, interview, 6.
18. Edwards-Madison, interview, 8.
19. Edwards-Madison, interview, 8.
20. Edwards-Madison, interview, 8.
21. Edwards-Madison, interview, 9.
22. "Lena Edwards Papers" Finding Aid 69 (2015), Howard University Moorland-Spingarn Research Center Collections, https://dh.howard.edu/cgi/viewcontent .cgi?referer=&httpsredir=1&article=1068&context=finaid_manu.
23. Leo Adam Biga, "Black Legacy Families, Installment I: The Metoyers," NOISE: North Omaha Information Support Everyone, last modified March 22, 2021, https:// www.noiseomaha.com/profiles/2021/3/22/uvdqrz1dch3vyf7s6ws2c405c308mg.
24. "Dr. Marie Metoyer (MD '51) Leaves Lasting Legacy."
25. Edwards-Madison, interview, 13.
26. "Marie S. Metoyer (1925–2020)," Black Heritage Trail of New Hampshire, https:// blackheritagetrailnh.org/marie-s-metoyer-1925–2020.
27. "Dr. Marie Metoyer (MD '51) Leaves Lasting Legacy"; "Marie S. Metoyer (1925–2020)."
28. Earl Morgan, "Jersey City Family the Gold Standard for African-American MDs," *Jersey Journal*, last modified January 16, 2019, https://www.nj.com/opinion/2016/12 /jersey_city_family_the_gold_standard_for_african-a.html.

CHAPTER 5: FINDING FULFILLMENT IN GIVING BACK

1. Edith Irby Jones, interview by Scott Lunsford, April 3, 2006, Pryor Center for Arkansas Oral and Visual History, Special Collections, University of Arkansas Libraries Arkansas Memories Project, 7, https://pryorcenter.uark.edu/projects

/Arkansas%20Memories/JONES-Edith-Irby/transcripts/TRANS-JONES-Edith
-Irby-Memories-20060403.pdf.

2. Jones, interview, 8.
3. Jones, interview, 17–18.
4. Jones, interview, 53.
5. Jones, interview, 57–58.
6. Jones, interview, 94.
7. Jones, interview, 99.
8. Richard Sandomir, "Edith Irby Jones, Barrier-Breaking Doctor in the South, Dies at 91," *New York Times*, July 23, 2019, https://www.nytimes.com/2019/07/23/obituaries/dr-edith-irby-jones-dead.html.
9. Jones, interview, 106.
10. Jones, interview, 108.
11. Jones, interview, 110.
12. Jones, interview, 110.
13. Jones, interview, 112.
14. Michelle Nevius and James Nevius, "Thurgood Marshall's Harlem," Inside the Apple: A Streetwise History of New York City, last modified August 30, 2012, http://blog.insidetheapple.net/2012/08/thurgood-marshalls-harlem.html; "Who's May Chinn?" Richard Allen Center for Culture and Art, http://www.raccaseaportsalon.com/raccaseaportsalon.com/Whos_May_Chinn.html; Charisse Burden-Stelly, "Radical Blackness and Mutual Comradeship at 409 Edgecombe," Black Perspectives, African American Intellectual History Society, last modified July 16, 2019, https://www.aaihs.org/radical-blackness-and-mutual-comradeship-at-409-edgecombe.
15. M. I. Douglass, "The Legacy of William Montague Cobb, MD, PhD (1904–1990)," *Journal of the National Medical Association* 84, no. 10 (1992): 885, https://www.ncbi.nlm.nih.gov/pmc/articles/PMC2571791/pdf/jnma00276-0081.pdf.
16. Jones, interview, 115.
17. Jones, interview, 115.
18. Jones, interview, 115.
19. Jones, interview, 116.
20. Jones, interview, 117.
21. Jones, interview, 118.
22. John Kirk, "The Legacy of William Harold Flowers: The Pine Bluff Attorney Made the NAACP Powerful in Arkansas," *Arkansas Times*, February 1, 2018, https://arktimes.com/news/cover-stories/2018/02/01/the-legacy-of-william-harold-flowers; "Meet Local Legend: Edith Irby Jones, M.D.," Local Legends: Celebrating America's Local Women Physicians, National Library of Medicine, https://wayback.archive-it.org/org-350/20190508153550/https://www.nlm.nih.gov/exhibition/locallegends/Biographies/Jones_Edith.html.
23. Jones, interview, 130.
24. Lauran Kerr-Healy, "Jones, Edith Mae Irby (1927–2019)," *Handbook of Texas Online*, Texas State Historical Association, last modified March 19, 2021, https://www.tshaonline.org/handbook/entries/jones-edith-mae-irby.
25. "Dr. Edith Irby Jones," Changing the Face of Medicine, National Library of Medicine, National Institutes of Health, last modified June 3, 2015, https://cfmedicine.nlm.nih.gov/physicians/biography_175.html.

26. Jeffrey D. Quinlan and Neil J. Murphy, "Cesarean Delivery: Counseling Issues and Complication Management," *American Family Physician* 91, no. 3 (February 1, 2015): 178–84, https://www.aafp.org/afp/2015/0201/p178.html.
27. "Working Together to Reduce Black Maternal Mortality," Office of Minority Health & Health Equity, Centers for Disease Control and Prevention, last modified April 9, 2021, https://www.cdc.gov/healthequity/features/maternal-mortality/index.html.
28. Jones, interview, 149.
29. "Dr. Edith Irby Jones (1927–2019): 2015 Inductee," Arkansas Women's Hall of Fame, https://www.arwomenshalloffame.com/edith-jones; Kerr-Healy, "Jones, Edith Mae Irby."
30. "Dr. Edith Irby Jones: 2015 Inductee."
31. Kerr-Healy, "Jones, Edith Mae Irby."
32. "Dr. Edith Irby Jones," Changing the Face of Medicine.
33. "Dr. Edith Irby Jones," Changing the Face of Medicine.

CHAPTER 6: YOU CAN'T BE WHAT YOU CAN'T SEE

1. M. Joycelyn Elders and David Chanoff, *Joycelyn Elders, M.D.: From Sharecropper's Daughter to Surgeon General of the United States* (New York: William Morrow, 1996), 11–12.
2. Joycelyn Elders, interview by Scott Lunsford, February 14, 2008, Pryor Center for Arkansas Oral and Visual History, Special Collections, University of Arkansas Libraries Arkansas Memories Project, 10, https://pryorcenter.uark.edu/interview .php?thisProject=Arkansas%20Memories&thisProfileURL=ELDERS-Joycelyn &displayName=&thisInterviewee=202.
3. Elders, Arkansas Memories Project interview, 39.
4. Elders, Arkansas Memories Project interview, 39-40.
5. Elders, Arkansas Memories Project interview, 40.
6. Elders, Arkansas Memories Project interview, 59.
7. Joycelyn Elders, interview by Crystal R. Emery, *Black Women in Medicine*, directed by Crystal R. Emery (West Haven, CT: URU the Right to Be, 2016), 2.
8. Elders, Arkansas Memories Project interview, 60.
9. Elders, *Black Women in Medicine* interview, 4.
10. Elders, Arkansas Memories Project interview, 63.
11. Elders, *Black Women in Medicine* interview, 6.
12. Elders, *Black Women in Medicine* interview, 1.
13. Elders, *Black Women in Medicine* interview, 8.
14. Elders and Chanoff, *Joycelyn Elders, M.D.*, 90.
15. Elders, *Black Women in Medicine* interview, 9–10.
16. Elders and Chanoff, *Joycelyn Elders, M.D.*, 103.
17. Elders and Chanoff, *Joycelyn Elders, M.D.*, 106.
18. Elders and Chanoff, *Joycelyn Elders, M.D.*, 108.
19. Elders and Chanoff, *Joycelyn Elders, M.D.*, 111.
20. Elders and Chanoff, *Joycelyn Elders, M.D.*, 112.
21. Elders and Chanoff, *Joycelyn Elders, M.D.*, 113.
22. Elders and Chanoff, *Joycelyn Elders, M.D.*, 114.
23. Elders and Chanoff, *Joycelyn Elders, M.D.*, 114.
24. Elders and Chanoff, *Joycelyn Elders, M.D.*, 223.

25. Elders and Chanoff, *Joycelyn Elders, M.D.*, 232.
26. Elders, Arkansas Memories Project interview, 123.
27. Elders and Chanoff, *Joycelyn Elders, M.D.*, 5, 281.
28. Elders and Chanoff, *Joycelyn Elders, M.D.*, 310.
29. Elders and Chanoff, *Joycelyn Elders, M.D.*, 5.
30. Carl M. Cannon, "Clinton Fires Surgeon General," *Baltimore Sun*, December 10, 1994, https://www.baltimoresun.com/news/bs-xpm-1994–12–10–1994344068 -story.html.
31. Elders, *Black Women in Medicine* interview, 1.

CHAPTER 7: HEALTHCARE IS A HUMAN RIGHT
1. "Dr. Marilyn Hughes Gaston," Changing the Face of Medicine, National Library of Medicine, National Institutes of Health, last modified June 3, 2015, https://cf medicine.nlm.nih.gov/physicians/biography_124.html.
2. Marilyn Gaston, interview by Crystal R. Emery, *Black Women in Medicine*, directed by Crystal R. Emery (West Haven, CT: URU the Right to Be, 2011), 3.
3. Gaston, interview, 3.
4. Gaston, interview, 3.
5. "Gaston," Changing the Face of Medicine.
6. Gaston, interview, 10.
7. Gaston, interview, 11.
8. Association of American Medical Colleges, *Diversity in the Physician Workforce: Facts & Figures 2006*, 21, https://www.aamc.org/system/files/reports/1/diversity inthephysicianworkforce-factsandfigures2006.pdf.
9. "About Us," Department of Public Health, City of Philadelphia, last updated June 4, 2020, https://www.phila.gov/departments/department-of-public-health/about -us; James Higgins, "Public Health," *The Encyclopedia of Greater Philadelphia*, Mid-Atlantic Regional Center for the Humanities, Rutgers University-Camden, https://philadelphiaencyclopedia.org/archive/public-health.
10. Gaston, interview, 4.
11. Gaston, interview, 4.
12. Association of American Medical Colleges, *Diversity in the Physician Workforce: Facts & Figures 2006*, 24.
13. "A Summing Up: Louis Lomax Interviews Malcolm X," Teachingamericanhistory .org, Ashbrook Center, Ashbrook University, accessed March 1, 2022, https:// teachingamericanhistory.org/document/a-summing-up-louis-lomax-interviews -malcolm-x.
14. Martin Luther King Jr., *Why We Can't Wait* (New York: Harper & Row, 1964), 19.
15. King, *Why We Can't Wait*, 20.
16. King, *Why We Can't Wait*, 20–21.
17. "History," Healthcare Connection, https://healthcare-connection.org/history.
18. Mark Curnutte, "Dolores Lindsay Became the Change She Sought 50 Years Ago in Lincoln Heights," *Cincinnati Enquirer*, November 22, 2017, https://www.cincinnati .com/story/news/2017/11/22/dolores-lindsay-became-change-she-sought-50-years -and-clinic-she-started-50-years-ago-lincoln-height/826441001.
19. Curnutte, "Dolores Lindsay Became the Change She Sought 50 Years Ago in Lincoln Heights."

20. "Sickle Cell Anemia," MayoClinic.org, last modified July 17, 2021, https://www
.mayoclinic.org/diseases-conditions/sickle-cell-anemia/symptoms-causes/syc
-20355876.

21. Dominique Bulgin, Paula Tanabe, and Coretta Jenerette, "Stigma of Sickle Cell
Disease: A Systematic Review," *Issues in Mental Health Nursing* 39, no. 8 (2018),
https://www.ncbi.nlm.nih.gov/pmc/articles/PMC6186193.

22. Jennifer Hodge, "Overcoming the Stigma of Sickle Cell Disease," Gethealthystay
healthy.com, Pfizer, February 27, 2020, https://www.gethealthystayhealthy.com
/articles/overcoming-the-stigma-of-sickle-cell-disease.

23. Gaston, interview, 17.

24. Jenny Gold, "Sickle Cell Patients Suffer Discrimination, Poor Care—And Shorter
Lives," Californiahealthline.org, Kaiser Health News, https://californiahealthline
.org/news/sickle-cell-patients-suffer-discrimination-poor-care-and-shorter-lives.

25. "Richard Nixon: Special Message to the Congress Proposing a National Health
Strategy," February 18, 1971, American Presidency Project, University of California,
Santa Barbara, https://www.presidency.ucsb.edu/documents/special-message-the
-congress-proposing-national-health-strategy.

26. Alondra Nelson, "Spin Doctors: The Politics of Sickle Cell Anemia," in *Body and
Soul: The Black Panther Party and the Fight Against Medical Discrimination* (Minneapolis: University of Minnesota Press, 2013).

27. Robert B. Scott, "Health Care Priority and Sickle Cell Anemia," *JAMA (Journal
of the American Medical Association)* 214, no. 4 (October 26, 1970): 731–34, https://
jamanetwork.com/journals/jama/article-abstract/357392.

28. Nelson, "Spin Doctors."

29. Mary Hulihan et al., "CDC Grand Rounds: Improving the Lives of Persons with
Sickle Cell Disease," *Morbidity and Mortality Weekly Report*, 66, no. 46 (November
24, 2017): 1269–71, https://www.cdc.gov/mmwr/volumes/66/wr/mm6646a2.htm.

30. Gaston, interview, 10.

31. Gaston, interview, 10.

32. Marilyn H. Gaston et al., "Prophylaxis with Oral Penicillin in Children with Sickle
Cell Anemia: A Randomized Trial," *New England Journal of Medicine* 314, no. 25
(June 19, 1986): 1593–99, https://pubmed.ncbi.nlm.nih.gov/3086721.

33. "Gaston," Changing the Face of Medicine.

CHAPTER 8: "I WILL NOT BE THE LAST"

1. Association of American Medical Colleges, *Diversity in the Physician Workforce:
Facts & Figures 2006*, 23.

2. Association of American Medical Colleges, *Diversity in the Physician Workforce:
Facts & Figures 2010*, 35, https://www.aamc.org/media/8046/download.

3. Association of American Medical Colleges, *Diversity in the Physician Workforce:
Facts & Figures 2006*, 24–26.

4. Association of American Medical Colleges, *Diversity in the Physician Workforce:
Facts & Figures 2006*, 23.

5. Association of American Medical Colleges, *Current Trends in Medical Education:
Facts & Figures 2016*, fig. 17, https://www.aamcdiversityfactsandfigures2016.org
/report-section/section-3/#figure-17.

6. Richard Nixon, press conference on drug abuse, June 17, 1971, Richard Nixon Presidential Library and Museum, https://www.nixonfoundation.org/2016/06 /26404; "Richard Nixon: Special Message to the Congress on Drug Abuse Prevention and Control," June 17, 1971, American Presidency Project, University of California, Santa Barbara, https://www.presidency.ucsb.edu/documents/special -message-the-congress-drug-abuse-prevention-and-control.

7. James Cullen, "The History of Mass Incarceration," Brennan Center for Justice, July 20, 2018, https://www.brennancenter.org/our-work/analysis-opinion/history -mass-incarceration.

8. American Civil Liberties Union, "Banking on Bondage: Private Prisons and Mass Incarceration," November 2, 2011, https://www.aclu.org/banking-bondage-private -prisons-and-mass-incarceration?redirect=prisoners-rights/banking-bondage -private-prisons-and-mass-incarceration.

9. Lipi Roy, "'It's My Calling to Change the Statistics': Why We Need More Black Female Physicians," *Forbes*, February 25, 2020, https://www.forbes.com/sites /lipiroy/2020/02/25/its-my-calling-to-change-the-statistics-why-we-need-more -black-female-physicians/?sh=2c51a35b56a5.

10. Association of American Medical Colleges, *Diversity in the Physician Workforce: Facts & Figures 2010*, 31; Association of American Medical Colleges, *Diversity in Medical Education: Facts & Figures 2012*, 30–32, https://www.aamc.org/media/9951 /download.

11. Madeline Will, "65 Years After 'Brown v. Board,' Where Are All the Black Educators?" *Education Week*, May 14, 2019, https://www.edweek.org/policy-politics/65 -years-after-brown-v-board-where-are-all-the-black-educators/2019/05.

12. Will, "65 Years After 'Brown v. Board.'"

13. Will, "65 Years After 'Brown v. Board.'"

14. John Rosales and Tim Walker, "The Racist Beginnings of Standardized Testing," New from NEA, National Education Association, March 20, 2021, https://www.nea .org/advocating-for-change/new-from-nea/racist-beginnings-standardized-testing.

15. Jacob Landers, "Improving Ethnic Distribution of New York City Pupils," May 1966, New York City Board of Education, https://files.eric.ed.gov/fulltext/ED011270.pdf.

16. "Claudia Lynn Thomas '71: Takeover of Main Building, 1969," Vassar Encyclopedia, https://www.vassar.edu/vcencyclopedia/interviews-reflections/claudia-lynn -thomas.html.

17. National Merit Scholarship Corporation, "Flashback Friday," September 14, 2018, https://www.nationalmerit.org/s/1758/blog.aspx?pgid=856&gid=2&cid=1381.

18. "NYS Scholarships for Academic Excellence," Higher Education Services Corporation, New York State, https://www.hesc.ny.gov/pay-for-college/financial-aid/types -of-financial-aid/nys-grants-scholarships-awards/nys-scholarships-for-academic -excellence.html, accessed March 1, 2022.

19. Claudia Lynn Thomas, interview by Roscoe C. Brown Jr., October 10, 2007, "African American Legends: Dr. Claudia Lynn Thomas," CUNY TV, https://tv.cuny .edu/show/africanamericanlegends/PR1009144.

20. Thomas, "African American Legends" interview.

21. Claudia Thomas, interview with Crystal R. Emery, *Black Women in Medicine*, directed by Crystal R. Emery (West Haven, CT: URU the Right to Be, 2016), 1.

22. Thomas, *Black Women in Medicine* interview, 4.
23. Thomas, "African American Legends" interview.
24. Thomas, *Black Women in Medicine* interview, 4.
25. "Ward by Ward: Hopkins Nurse Leaves Legacy of Desegregation," April 5, 2010, On the Pulse, Johns Hopkins Nursing, https://magazine.nursing.jhu.edu/2010/04 /ward-by-ward-2.
26. Thomas, *Black Women in Medicine* interview, 4.
27. Thomas, *Black Women in Medicine* interview, 4.
28. Thomas, *Black Women in Medicine* interview, 4.
29. Thomas, *Black Women in Medicine* interview, 4.
30. Thomas, *Black Women in Medicine* interview, 6.
31. Thomas, *Black Women in Medicine* interview, 7.
32. "Claudia L. Thomas, M.D.: The Artistry of Orthopaedics," Unovahealth.com, https://www.unovahealth.com/ortho/claudia-l-thomas-m-d, accessed May 7, 2022.
33. Thomas, *Black Women in Medicine* interview, 6.
34. Globe Newswire, "Claudia Thomas, MD: A Pioneer on Two Fronts," news release, March 6, 2008, https://www.globenewswire.com/en/news-release/2008/03/06 /1234494/0/en/Claudia-Thomas-MD-A-Pioneer-on-Two-Fronts.html.
35. Peter Pollack, "Claudia Thomas, MD, Wins 2008 Diversity Award," April 1, 2008, AAOS Now, American Academy of Orthopaedic Surgeons, https://www.aaos.org /aaosnow/2008/apr/youraaos/youraaos4.
36. Pollack, "Claudia Thomas, MD, Wins 2008 Diversity Award."
37. Bonnie S. Mason, "The Power of Mentoring," *Nth Dimensions* (blog), January 8, 2019, http://www.nthdimensions.org/blog/2019/1/8/the-power-of-mentoring.
38. Mason, "The Power of Mentoring."
39. "About," *Nth Dimensions*, http://www.nthdimensions.org/about-nthdimensions.
40. "About," Bonnie Simpson Mason's website, http://www.drbonniemason.com /about, accessed April 8, 2022.
41. Molly A. Day, Jessell M. Owens, and Lindsey S. Caldwell, "Breaking Barriers: A Brief Overview of Diversity in Orthopedic Surgery," *Iowa Orthopaedic Journal* 39, no. 1 (2019): 1–5, https://www.ncbi.nlm.nih.gov/pmc/articles/PMC6604536.
42. Thomas, *Black Women in Medicine* interview, 11.
43. "Dr. Claudia L. Thomas Wed to Maxwell Carty," *New York Times*, August 25, 1985, https://www.nytimes.com/1985/08/25/style/dr-claudia-l-thomas-wed-to-maxwell -carty.html.
44. Ryan Park, "Why So Many Young Doctors Work Such Awful Hours," *The Atlantic*, February 21, 2017, https://www.theatlantic.com/business/archive/2017/02 /doctors-long-hours-schedules/516639.
45. "The ACGME's Approach to Limit Resident Duty Hours 12 Months After Implementation: A Summary of Achievements," Accreditation Council for Graduate Medical Education, https://www.acgme.org/globalassets/PFAssets/Publications Papers/dh_dutyhoursummary2003-04.pdf, accessed May 7, 2022; Anupam B. Jena et al., "Exposing Physicians to Reduced Residency Work Hours Did Not Adversely Affect Patient Outcomes After Residency," *Health Affairs* 33, no. 10 (October 2014): 1832–40, https://www.healthaffairs.org/doi/10.1377/hlthaff.2014.0318?url_ver=Z39 .88-2003&rfr_id=ori:rid:crossref.org&rfr_dat=cr_pub%3dpubmed.

CHAPTER 9: CRUSADING FOR PUBLIC HEALTH

1. Association of American Medical Colleges, *U.S. Medical School Deans by Dean Type and Sex*, last modified January 2022, https://www.aamc.org/data-reports /faculty-institutions/interactive-data/us-medical-school-deans-dean-type-and-sex.

2. "About the President and Dean: Valerie Montgomery Rice, MD, FACOG," Morehouse School of Medicine, https://www.msm.edu/Administration/office_president /about_the_president.php, accessed March 1, 2022; "Home Page," Charles R. Drew University of Medicine and Science, accessed March 1, 2022, https://www.cdrewu .edu/com.

3. Risa Lavizzo-Mourey, former president and CEO of the Robert Wood Johnson Foundation, in discussion with the author, June 2021.

4. Lavizzo-Mourey, in discussion with the author.

5. Lavizzo-Mourey, in discussion with the author.

6. Lavizzo-Mourey, in discussion with the author.

7. Lavizzo-Mourey, in discussion with the author.

8. Irene Monroe, "Boston's Racist Past Haunts Its Present," WGBH.org, April 10, 2017, https://www.wgbh.org/news/2017/04/10/how-we-live/bostons-racist-past -haunts-its-present.

9. "1972, Morgan v. Hennigan: Racial Segregation Abolished in Boston Public Schools," *Long Road to Justice: The African American Experience in the Massachusetts Courts*, permanent exhibition installed in the Edward W. Brooke Courthouse, Boston, in 2018, http://www.longroadtojustice.org/topics/education/morgan- hennigan.php, accessed March 1, 2022.

10. "Violence Erupts in Boston over Desegregation Busing," This Day in History: September 12, 1974, History.com, last modified September 12, 2019, https://www .history.com/this-day-in-history/violence-in-boston-over-racial-busing.

11. "Biography: Dr. Alvin Poussaint," The History Makers, https://www.thehistory makers.org/biography/dr-alvin-poussaint-39, accessed April 8, 2022.

12. M. R. F. Buckley, "Making History: Dr. Alvin Poussaint Reflects on a Lifetime of Achievement," News & Research, Harvard Medical School, May 16, 2019, https:// hms.harvard.edu/news/making-history-0.

13. Risa Lavizzo-Mourey, interview with Joan Ilacqua, May 2, 2016, Perspectives of Change: The Story of Civil Rights, Diversity, Inclusion, and Access to Education, HMS and HSDM Collection, Center for the History of Medicine, Francis A. Countway Library of Medicine, 7–8, https://collections.countway.harvard.edu /onview/items/show/18137.

14. Uche Blackstock, "Why Black Doctors Like Me Are Leaving Faculty Positions in Academic Medical Centers," *STAT News*, January 16, 2020, https://www.statnews .com/2020/01/16/black-doctors-leaving-faculty-positions-academic-medical-centers.

15. Roy, "'It's My Calling'"; Sophie Balzora, "When the Minority Tax Is Doubled: Being Black and Female in Academic Medicine," *Nature Reviews Gastroenterology & Hepatology* 18, vol. 1 (September 22, 2020), https://www.nature.com/articles /s41575-020-00369-2.

16. "Background/History," Association for Academic Minority Physicians, https:// www.aampinc.org/history, accessed March 1, 2022.

17. Lavizzo-Mourey, in discussion with the author.

18. Lavizzo-Mourey, in discussion with the author.

19. Lavizzo-Mourey, in discussion with the author.

20. Sandra Salmans, "In Person; Treating Health Care," *New York Times*, October 6, 2002, https://www.nytimes.com/2002/10/06/nyregion/in-person-treating-health-care.html.

21. Kamala Harris, "Watch Kamala Harris's First Speech to the Nation as Vice President-Elect," CNBC Television, November 7, 2020, available on YouTube, 11:30, https://www.youtube.com/watch?v=2VdwMNexBHc.

22. Susan Loyer, "Search Is on for New CEO of Robert Wood Johnson Foundation," *My Central Jersey*, September 26, 2016, https://www.mycentraljersey.com/story/life/wellness/2016/09/26/search-new-ceo-robert-wood-johnson-foundation/90367768.

23. Cynthia Ogden and Margaret Carroll, "Prevalence of Obesity Among Children and Adolescents: United States, Trends 1963–1965 Through 2007–2008," National Center for Health Statistics, Centers for Disease Control and Prevention, last modified November 6, 2015, https://www.cdc.gov/nchs/data/hestat/obesity_child_07_08/obesity_child_07_08.htm.

24. Cynthia L. Ogden et al., "Prevalence of Obesity and Trends in Body Mass Index Among US Children and Adolescents, 1999–2010," *Journal of the American Medical Association* 307, no. 5 (January 17, 2012): 483–90, https://pubmed.ncbi.nlm.nih.gov/22253364.

25. Cynthia L. Ogden et al., "Prevalence of Childhood and Adult Obesity in the United States, 2011–2012," *Journal of the American Medical Association* 311, no. 8 (February 26, 2014): 806–14, https://www.ncbi.nlm.nih.gov/pmc/articles/PMC4770258.

26. Loyer, "Search Is on for New CEO of Robert Wood Johnson Foundation."

27. Loyer, "Search Is on for New CEO of Robert Wood Johnson Foundation."

28. Lavizzo-Mourey, in discussion with the author.

IMAGE CREDITS

p. 16: Dr. May Chinn: Courtesy of *Harlem World Magazine*

p. 38: Dr. Dorothy Ferebee: Courtesy of Moorland-Springarn Research Center, Howard University

p. 60: Dr. Lena Edwards: Courtesy of the US National Library of Medicine

p. 80: Dr. Edith Irby Jones: Courtesy of the US National Library of Medicine

p. 104: US Surgeon General Dr. Joycelyn Elders: Courtesy of the University of Arkansas Medical Sciences Historical Research Center

p. 128: Dr. Marilyn Hughes Gaston: Courtesy of the Maryland Governor's Press Office

p. 152: Dr. Claudia Thomas: Courtesy of Dr. Claudia Thomas

p. 172: Dr. Risa Lavizzo-Mourey: Courtesy of Dr. Risa Lavizzo-Mourey

INDEX

academic medicine, 181, 186

Accreditation Council for Graduate Medical Education, "duty hour" restrictions, 170

affirmative action, 135, 178–79, 183–84

"African American," as a term, xiv

African American physicians: decreasing numbers, 154–55; and the leadership/contributions of black women, xiv, xvi, 174, 196; limited numbers of, 153–54; limits placed on, 20; and mass incarceration, 153–55; number of women, 17, 154–55; obstacles faced by, 8, 17–21, 32, , 41–49, 62–63, 70–71, 93–95, 117, 180, 183, 194–96; quotas, 66. *See also* medical training; misogyny; racism; *and individual doctors*

African Americans: educational inequities, 49–50, 157–58; health issues faced by, 35, 54–55, 133, 140–41; healthcare inequities, 21, 98–100, 108–9; impacts of mass incarceration, 154; housing inequities, 67; responses to the *Brown* decision, 156–57; stereotypes about intelligence/laziness, viii–x, xiii, xv, 108, 163, 179, 196; successful artists among, 27. *See also* medical training; racism; sickle cell disease

African Free School No. 2, New York City, 2–3

African Meeting House, Boston, 9–10

Afro-American Society, Vassar College, 159–60

Agency of Health Care Policy and Research, 188

allopathic medicine, xii–xiii, 1–2, 4, 12–13, 17–18, 28, 78

Alpha Kappa Alpha Sorority, 53–55, 58, 186

ambulances, Ferebee's work on board, 49

American Academy of Orthopaedic Surgeons (AAOS), Diversity Award, 167

American Food for Peace Council, 56

American Medical Association (AMA), 18–19, 137, 144

Arkansas Department of Health, 121–22

Arkansas State Press, support for Jones's medical education, 90

Arthur, Mary, 96

Association of Academic Minority Physicians (AAMP), 187

Bates, Daisy and L. C., 90–91

Baylor College of Medicine Affiliated Hospitals, Houston, Irby Jones's internship, 101

Beaty, James, 167

"Beyond Health Care" report (Robert Wood Johnson Foundation), 193

"black," as a term, xiv

Black Panther Party, 144

Blackwell, Elizabeth, 5–8

blood transfusions, direct, 35

Booker, Bob, 97

A Book of Medical Discourses: In Two Parts (Crumpler), 13, 15